Education for Occupational Therapy in Health Care: Strategies for the New Millennium

Education for Occupational Therapy in Health Care: Strategies for the New Millennium has been co-published simultaneously as *Occupational Therapy in Health Care*, Volume 15, Numbers 1/2 2001.

The *Occupational Therapy in Health Care* Monographic "Separates"

Below is a list of "separates," which in serials librarianship means a special issue simultaneously published as a special journal issue or double-issue *and* as a "separate" hardbound monograph. (This is a format which we also call a "DocuSerial.")

"Separates" are published because specialized libraries or professionals may wish to purchase a specific thematic issue by itself in a format which can be separately cataloged and shelved, as opposed to purchasing the journal on an on-going basis. Faculty members may also more easily consider a "separate" for classroom adoption.

"Separates" are carefully classified separately with the major book jobbers so that the journal tie-in can be noted on new book order slips to avoid duplicate purchasing.

You may wish to visit Haworth's website at . . .

http://www.HaworthPress.com

. . . to search our online catalog for complete tables of contents of these separates and related publications.

You may also call 1-800-HAWORTH (outside US/Canada: 607-722-5857), or Fax: 1-800-895-0582 (outside US/Canada: 607-771-0012), or e-mail at:

getinfo@haworthpressinc.com

Education for Occupational Therapy in Health Care: Strategies for the New Millennium, edited by Patricia Crist, PhD, OTR/L, FAOTA, and Marjorie Scaffa, PhD, OTR/L, FAOTA (Vol. 15, No. 1/2, 2001). *"PROVIDES TRULY IMAGINATIVE IDEAS for preparing the practitioners of the near future–and not a moment too soon! It is easy to see that these authors have been outstanding clinicians . . . they put their OT skills to work in creating these unique learning-by-doing educational packages. Especially exciting are the clever ways in which alternative sites and programs are used to provide fieldwork experiences."* (Nedra P. Gillette, MEd, OTR, ScD (Hon), Director, Institute for the Study of Occupation and Health, American Occupational Therapy Foundation)

Community for Occupational Therapy Education and Practice, edited by Beth P. Velde, PhD, OTR/L, and Peggy Prince Wittman, EdD, OTR/L, FAOTA (Vol. 13, No. 3/4, 2001). *"Introduces the concept of community-based practice in non-traditional settings. Whether one is concerned with wellness and the aging process or with debilitating situations, injuries, or diseases such as homelessness, AIDS, or multiple sclerosis, this collection details the process of moving forward."* (Scott D. McPhee, DrPH, OT, FAOTA, Associate Dean and Chair, School of Occupational Therapy, Belmont University, Nashville, Tennessee)

Education for Occupational Therapy in Health Care: Strategies for the New Millennium

Patricia Crist, PhD
Marjorie Scaffa, PhD
Editors

Education for Occupational Therapy in Health Care: Strategies for the New Millennium has been co-published simultaneously as *Occupational Therapy in Health Care*, Volume 15, Numbers 1/2 2001.

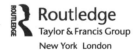

Routledge
Taylor & Francis Group
New York London

This edition published 2012 by Routledge

Routledge
Taylor & Francis Group
711 Third Avenue
New York, NY 10017

Routledge
Taylor & Francis Group
2 Park Square
Milton Park, Abingdon
Oxon OX14 4RN

Education for Occupational Therapy in Health Care: Strategies for the New Millennium has been co-published simultaneously as *Occupational Therapy in Health Care*™, Volume 15, Numbers 1/2 2001.

The development, preparation, and publication of this work has been undertaken with great care. However, the publisher, employees, editors, and agents of The Haworth Press and all imprints of The Haworth Press, Inc., including The Haworth Medical Press® and Pharmaceutical Products Press®, are not responsible for any errors contained herein or for consequences that may ensue from use of materials or information contained in this work. Opinions expressed by the author(s) are not necessarily those of The Haworth Press, Inc. With regard to case studies, identities and circumstances of individuals discussed herein have been changed to protect confidentiality. Any resemblance to actual persons, living or dead, is entirely coincidental.

Cover design by Thomas J. Mayshock, Jr.

Library of Congress Cataloging-in-Publication Data

Education for occupational therapy in health care : strategies for the new millennium / Patricia Crist, Majorie Scaffa, editors.
    p. ; cm.
"Co-published simultaneously as: Occupational therapy in health care, volume 15, numbers 1/2 2002."
Includes bibliographical references and index.
    ISBN 0-7890-1686-9 (hard : alk. paper) – ISBN 0-7890-1687-7 (pbk. : alk. paper)
    1. Occupational therapy–Study and teaching.
    [DNLM: 1. Occupational Therapy–education. WB 18 E238 2002] I. Crist, Patricia A. Hickerson. II. Scaffa, Marjorie E. III. Occupational therapy in health care.
RM735.42 .E383 2002
615.8'515'071–dc21

2002002356

Education for Occupational Therapy in Health Care: Strategies for the New Millennium

CONTENTS

FIELDWORK EDUCATION

OCCUPATIONAL THERAPY ASSISTANT EDUCATION

ACADEMIC LEADERSHIP

STUDENT DEVELOPMENT

COMMENTARY ON EDUCATION

ABOUT THE EDITORS

Patricia Crist, PhD, OTR/L, FAOTA, is Founding Chair and Professor in the Department of Occupational Therapy at Duquesne University in Pittsburgh, Pennsylvania. Dr. Crist has produced numerous publications. Among them, she is co-editor of *Innovations in OT Education* and co-author of the self-study *Meeting the Fieldwork Challenge*. She also writes the popular "Fieldwork Issue" column for *OT Advance*. Dr. Crist has completed numerous scholarly works regarding fieldwork education, mental health interventions, parents with disabilities, and research. Currently, she is on the Board of Directors of the National Certification Board of Occupational Therapy.

Marjorie Scaffa, PhD, OTR/L, FAOTA, is Associate Professor and Chairperson of the Department of Occupational Therapy at the University of South Alabama in Mobile, and of the OT therapy program she founded in 1993. She is the editor of the book *Occupational Therapy in Community-Based Practice Settings*. Dr. Scaffa has worked in a number of clinical and community settings, including inpatient rehabilitation, home health, long-term care, hospice, alcohol/drug prevention and treatment programs, and community mental health. She served as an editorial board member for the *American Journal of Occupational Therapy* from 1997-1999 and is a Fellow of the American Occupational Therapy Association.

A Message from the Editors

We are very pleased to be able to bring this special volume on Occupational Therapy (OT) education in the new millennium to fruition. Our thanks go to Anne Dickerson and Susan Kaplan, Editors of *Occupational Therapy in Health Care,* who invited us to edit this special collection on education. They clearly see the need and value for educators to share scholarship regarding academic and fieldwork education. They have distinguished themselves as advocates for occupational therapy education.

The overarching theme of this book is CHANGE, including changes in health care delivery, in reimbursement, in OT practice, in professional preparation, and in accreditation standards. We can choose to view change as threatening and negative or as an opportunity for growth and revitalization. All of the contributors to this special collection have chosen to embrace change and creatively forge new pathways in education and practice.

All contributions were peer reviewed by an editorial board consisting of invited and ongoing OTHC editorial board members. We thank the following individuals for their service in this capacity:

Anne Blakeney	Martha Branson Banks	Alfred Bracciano
Janet Delany	Elizabeth Depoy	Linda Duncombe
Lynn Hazard	Elizabeth Kanny	Ellen Kolodner
Scott McPhee	Anne Neville-Jan	Barbara Schell
Janette Schkade	Ellen Spergel	Perri Stern
Louise Thibodaux	Barbara Veigl	Donna Whitehouse

The manuscripts in this book are divided into five categories: instructional methodology, fieldwork education, occupational therapy assistant education, academic leadership, and student development. Some of the selections are designated as "brief" or "new," meaning that the ideas or concepts presented are

[Haworth co-indexing entry note]: "A Message from the Editors." Crist, Patricia, and Marjorie Scaffa. Co-published simultaneously in *Occupational Therapy in Health Care* (The Haworth Press, Inc.) Vol. 15, No. 1/2, 2001, pp. 1-2; and: *Education for Occupational Therapy in Health Care: Strategies for the New Millennium* (eds: Patricia Crist, and Marjorie Scaffa) The Haworth Press, Inc., 2001, pp. 1-2. Single or multiple copies of this article are available for a fee from The Haworth Document Delivery Service [1-800-HAWORTH, 9:00 a.m. - 5:00 p.m. (EST). E-mail address: getinfo@haworthpressinc.com].

interesting and provocative, but may not yet be fully developed or evaluated. Other selections are full manuscripts that include educational methods or strategies that have been evaluated and further refined. Some of the topics addressed by the contributors include interactive reasoning, collaborative learning, the influence of learning styles, developing research competencies, understanding disability in context, establishing community partnerships, and creating new job possibilities. All provide some form of outcomes evidence that we believe is essential to validate educational premises and demonstrate the hypothesized or projected impact. We must ensure "best practices" in education as well as practice through being scholars of our instructional methods and educational approaches.

In addition, we have asked a number of leaders in the profession to provide commentaries on education. These include Charlotte Brasic Royeen, Commission on Education Chair; Nedra Gillette, American Occupational Therapy Foundation (AOTF); Barbara Kornblau, American Occupational Therapy Association (AOTA) President; Joseph Isaacs and Doris Gordon, AOTA National Office; and L. Randy Strickland, National Board for Certification in Occupational Therapy President.

The focus on change and a paradigm shift in education resonates throughout these commentaries. Royeen describes changes in education, including the integration of instructional technology with traditional methods, interdisciplinary collaboration through service-learning, and a shift from a focus on teaching to an emphasis on learning. Isaacs and Gordon advocate for a "cultural change" in the profession, moving from a state of dependency to one of "greater self-sufficiency, creativity, leadership and . . . advocacy." Kornblau echoes the need to develop independent, creative, and entrepreneurial practitioners who are willing to establish new venues in the community in which to provide OT services. Gillette calls on educators to become collaborators with AOTF in the work of the Institute for the Study of Occupation and Health and to expand the focus of the profession to include the health of populations at the societal level. Strickland overviews NBCOT processes to better understand the relationship within our educational and professional systems.

As Editors, we are impressed with the commitment, creativity, and vision that our leaders and educators bring to this special volume. We hope that the reader will be inspired and empowered to develop new volumes, methods, and approaches for OT Education in the New Millennium.

Patricia Crist, PhD, OTR/L, FAOTA
Marjorie Scaffa, PhD, OTR/L, FAOTA

Disability in Context:
A Community-Based Learning Experience

Sherry Borcherding, MA, OTR/L
Diana Baldwin, MA, OTR/L, FAOTA

Sherry Borcherding is Clinical Instructor at the University of Missouri-Columbia, where she teaches Disability in Context, Foundations of Healthcare, Health Care Delivery, and Loss and Disability. Sherry earned her BS with honors in Occupational Therapy at Texas Woman's University, and her MA in Education at George Peabody College, Nashville, TN. Before joining the faculty at the University of Missouri, she worked in ten different practice settings, bringing a rich clinical experience to her teaching duties. Her book, *A Documentation Manual for Writing SOAP Notes in Occupational Therapy*, is used in universities nationwide to teach documentation skills.

Diana Baldwin has been Chair of the Department of Occupational Therapy at the University of Missouri-Columbia for the past 15 years. She also teaches Research and Community Needs Assessment. Diana received her BS from Texas Woman's University and her MA from the University of Missouri-Kansas City. Her activity in the Missouri AgrAbility Project involves presenting statewide and nationally. She has received the Lindy Boggs Award in recognition of her service to enhance the appreciation and understanding of occupational therapy by elected and appointed officials.

Address correspondence to the authors at: Occupational Therapy Curriculum, 407 Lewis Hall, University of Missouri, Columbia, MO 65211 (E-mail: Borcherdings @health.missouri.edu) or (E-mail: Baldwind@health.missouri.edu).

[Haworth co-indexing entry note]: "Disability in Context: A Community-Based Learning Experience." Borcherding, Sherry, and Diana Baldwin. Co-published simultaneously in *Occupational Therapy in Health Care* (The Haworth Press, Inc.) Vol. 15, No. 1/2, 2001, pp. 3-12; and: *Education for Occupational Therapy in Health Care: Strategies for the New Millennium* (eds: Patricia Crist, and Marjorie Scaffa) The Haworth Press, Inc., 2001, pp. 3-12. Single or multiple copies of this article are available for a fee from The Haworth Document Delivery Service [1-800-HAWORTH, 9:00 a.m. - 5:00 p.m. (EST). E-mail address: getinfo@ haworthpressinc.com].

SUMMARY. This article describes a course in disability awareness that integrates didactic content with community-based Level 1 fieldwork experience. Course content includes the experience of disability, effective writing skills, peer review, interviewing techniques, and therapeutic relationships. In home and community settings, students interview and observe volunteers who have disabilities. In a teaching role, the volunteer exposes the student to resources utilized and barriers faced by a person with a disability living independently in the community. Professional documentation skills are developed through written assignments. This experiential course provides the opportunity for students to recognize the impact of dysfunction on human occupation and gain an appreciation of each individual's ability and responsibility for self-determination. *[Article copies available for a fee from The Haworth Document Delivery Service: 1-800-HAWORTH. E-mail address: <getinfo@haworthpressinc.com> Website: <http://www.HaworthPress.com> © 2001 by The Haworth Press, Inc. All rights reserved.]*

KEYWORDS. Fieldwork, community-based, disability

As the field of occupational therapy moves toward inclusion of less traditional work settings, community-based fieldwork placements become a very appealing option (Rydeen, Kautzmann, Cowan, & Benzing, 1995). These placements provide students with experiences that enhance their learning without overtaxing the already short supply of fieldwork sites. The PEW Commission report (1992) predicted a shift to home and community health interventions and the need for educational programs to prepare graduates for this changing practice setting. At the University of Missouri (MU), *Disability in Context* is a community fieldwork placement that provides a client-centered view of disabling conditions. As described in Table 1, the course objectives are designed to teach the interaction of the person-environment-occupation relationship as described by Law (1998). The student is exposed to a consumer model of self-determination based on motivation and choice (Bowen, 1996) for the purpose of learning to appreciate the context of the environment and personal life of someone who lives with a disabling condition. This learning experience occurs prior to the student becoming focused on occupational therapy interventions. The philosophy of the MU curriculum emphasizes empowerment and transformation as well as adaptation in adjusting to life where a disability is present. This concept of emphasizing a person's use of his/her individual strengths and resources within his/her own context is embodied

TABLE 1. *Disability in Context* Course Objectives

The student will be able to:

1. Demonstrate the ability to establish meaningful and comfortable relationships with persons experiencing cross-disabilities by:
    Demonstrating principles of good interviewing skills in practicing with classmates
    Meeting regularly with a volunteer who has a disability to establish rapport
    Administering a series of interview/assessment instruments to gain understanding
    of the volunteer's lifestyle, roles, and occupational choices
    Discussing characteristics of helping relationships as different from social relationships

2. Recognize the impact of disability on human occupation by:
    Observing how a person with a disability carries out daily living functions
    Analyzing internal and external adaptations made by a person with a disability living
    independently in the community
    Evaluating the response of the community to a person with a disability
    Assessing the roles and lifestyle of a person with a disability
    Using the peer review process to recognize the impact of a variety of different kinds
    of disabilities

3. Identify community resources and methods of accessing resources available for the disabled by:
    Describing the services discussed by guest speakers and how to access these
    Relating needs and problems discussed by disabled guest speakers to the services available
    in the community

4. Evaluate how a person with a disability would benefit from OT services by:
    Proposing a plan for OT services for the assigned volunteer
    Peer reviewing two additional plans for other disability areas

5. Demonstrate critical thinking skills and problem solving skills by:
    Peer reviewing papers on 8 volunteers having a variety of disabilities
    Analyzing the function and value of support groups and presenting this to class
    Setting goals for self for this experience and evaluating the outcome

throughout the curriculum (Department of Occupational Therapy, 1998). This course is the first of nine level I fieldwork placements in a variety of community and clinical settings.

Besides providing a community-based fieldwork experience, *Disability in Context* is intended to teach disability awareness. In the MU curriculum, as in many others across the country, there has existed the dilemma of how to expose students to the experience of disability. The placement with volunteers who have disabilities allows students to form a relationship with the volunteer and to see disability from the point of view of the person who is living with it successfully, before becoming enmeshed in an allopathic medical system that sees disability from quite a different perspective. Using the framework of the ICIDH-2 (World Health Organization, 2000), the student learns to view the volunteer's functioning level and capacity by assessing environmental and personal factors. Students are introduced to the independent living paradigm, or the idea that disability is a problem within society rather than a problem within the person. This is an idea long promoted by people with disabilities but not commonly held by rehabilitation professionals (Smart, 2001). The assignments require the student to identify the volunteer's problem solving skills and ability to achieve goals as an introduction to the concepts of client-centered therapy (McColl, Gerein, & Valentine, 1997). This community-based fieldwork course exposes the student to the complexities of the community and the relationship of occupation to functioning described by Fasio (2000). The student gains an understanding of community within the context of a disability.

Without regard to the kind of disability present, volunteers are selected for a desire to volunteer their time and a willingness to interact with the students. Volunteers have physical disabilities, mental illness, and developmental disabilities. Families who have children with disabilities also participate. Families with children who have disabilities teach students about the demands therapy can make on family life. Adults with visible disabilities teach students about public reaction to people who look different. Under the current accreditation standards (Accreditation Council for Occupational Therapy Education [ACOTE], 1998), students are asked to "understand the effects of health, disability, disease process, and traumatic injury to the individual within the context of family and society" (Section B.2.4.7). Students participate in the daily lives and activities of the volunteer, e.g., going to dance lessons with a child who has Down syndrome or visiting the psychiatric unit of the hospital to visit a volunteer who has suddenly been hospitalized. In the community, the student might eat in a restaurant with someone who cannot feed herself or use public transportation with someone who is trying to maneuver a wheelchair safely onto a city bus whose ramp does not quite touch the ground.

Class size averages 30 students, with one instructor. Students sign a confidentiality statement that applies to all settings, and are provided liability coverage through the University of Missouri Medical School liability policy. Students meet weekly for lecture and discussion as described in Table 2. Guest speakers and videotapes are also used to increase the breadth of the material. The majority of the speakers have disabilities. This is a reversal of the students' expected role of giving to or teaching those who live with disabling conditions. Class time is also used to provide the students with a forum for discussing their experiences and being actively engaged with the course content. The topic of interviewing, for example, is completed prior to meeting with the student's assigned volunteer. Students read a chapter from *Patient Practitioner Interaction* (Davis, 1998) on effective interviewing. They are asked questions about the content of the chapter, which encourages actually completing the reading assignment. The concept of open-ended questions is discussed in more detail with student-generated examples. In class, students in groups of three practice

TABLE 2. *Disability in Context* Course Format

Description
The course offers a beginning exposure to persons experiencing a variety of physical or mental disabilities, including families of children who have disabilities. It is intended to help students become sensitive to persons facing serious disabilities, to become comfortable interacting with such persons, and to see the person rather than only the disability.

Fieldwork Assignment
Students will be assigned to community volunteers with whom they will spend a minimum of 12 hours. There are assignments to be completed with the volunteer, and each assignment will result in a short paper. The student will be assigned to a volunteer and will be responsible for contacting the volunteer and arranging to meet with him/her and complete the assignment. One assignment will be due every other week at the time of seminar. Students will also attend support groups in the community and report on these in class.

Course Structure
Lecture topics will cover interviewing, therapeutic relationships, effective documentation, peer reviewing, "people-first" language, the Americans with Disabilities Act, rights and needs of people with disabilities, and services available. Seminar will be used to become acquainted with a wide variety of persons having disabilities as well as to develop skills in group interaction, critical thinking, problem solving, and peer review.

interviews, with the third person assisting the interviewer in using open-ended questions. Students are asked to write open-ended questions they might use in their first interview with their volunteer.

Each student is assigned to a volunteer for the course of the semester, and spends a minimum of 12 hours with the volunteer over five or more visits as described in Table 2. Each student interviews his/her assigned volunteer at least five times, using specific instruments each time to assess occupational performance. Instruments are chosen for their ease of use by inexperienced students and for their ability to provide information about occupational performance in persons who are beyond the stage of needing treatment in occupational therapy. The Occupational Questionnaire (Smith, Kielhofner, & Watts, 1986) is used for all volunteers, along with the Role Checklist (Oakley, 1982). The students are enrolled concurrently in a course on occupational performance and administer these instruments to themselves in class prior to using them with a volunteer. Using the Model of Human Occupation (Kielhofner, 1995), the assignments direct the student in assessing the volunteer's perspective on occupation and his/her motivation that influences the roles and habits assumed by the volunteer. Lefkovitz's Accessibility Evaluation of the home is used if the volunteer has a physical disability (Trombly & Versluys, 1989) along with a self-report of daily living activities. Children are assessed using a parent questionnaire about sensory motor development and a faculty-compiled developmental evaluation. Volunteers who have a mental illness complete a faculty-developed assessment of non-physical barriers to occupational functioning and a graphic representation of relationships.

In order to study public reaction to disability and accessibility issues, the volunteer and the student engage in a community outing, using whatever form of transportation that volunteer ordinarily uses. Students write a series of papers that replicate assessment reports used in occupational therapy, including recommendations regarding what occupational therapy might have to offer the volunteer. The papers allow the student to "exhibit the ability to analyze tasks relative to performance areas, performance components, and performance contexts" (ACOTE, 1998, B.2.8). Attitudes toward people with disability are explored, and often are changed through this experience, as evidenced by the students' comments in class and their evaluation of the course.

Professional writing skills are emphasized, particularly writing from a value-neutral perspective and from the client's point of view (Borcherding, 2000). Students are taught the difference between assessing the data and judging the patient. For example, early in the course a student might write an assessment stating "MC is a courageous woman who has struggled valiantly to overcome her mental illness." Later in the course the student might write, "MC's responses to the Role Checklist suggest that she has made several successful adaptations to her mental illness." This is a distinction that is crucial to professional documentation. There is an emphasis on identifying patterns found in the data. For example, a student comparing the results of the Role Checklist and the Occupational Questionnaire might write, "Consistencies were found between the results of the Role Checklist and the Occupational Questionnaire. The activities DH spoke of in his Occupational Questionnaire showed high personal causation, value and interest, and satisfied the roles he found valuable." Through these assignments, the students begin their clinical reasoning in the beginning semester of the occupational therapy curriculum by making sense of the data, recognizing patterns, understanding the situation, considering different possibilities, and making a recommendation that is realistic to the volunteer's situation (Barnes & Evenson, 2000). This course is credentialed as a campus writing intensive course, which requires opportunities to rewrite each paper to incorporate suggestions for improvement.

The course also provides an opportunity for peer review, a cooperative learning strategy for peer editing (Johnson, Johnson, & Smith, 1991). Peer review is a skill that has several professional applications. Reviewing the documentation of a peer is becoming more important as outcomes are scrutinized by payers. In addition, providing feedback on another person's work in a tactful, supportive, helpful way teaches skills that will become important in the supervisory responsibilities the student will assume as an occupational therapist. A rubric developed for peer review covers 17 items that are considered important in professional writing. Some of these items are essential with no points awarded for their inclusion, e.g., the paper must be typed, must follow the correct format, and must respect the volunteer's confidentiality. Other items under the headings of critical thinking, clarity and organization, professionalism, and mechanics of writing are rated from unsatisfactory to gold-star by the peer reviewers. Points are assigned by the instructor based on the students' ratings. Unsatisfactory items receive no credit, satisfactory items receive half credit, above satisfactory items receive full credit, and gold-star items receive extra credit. Students are evaluated on their ability to peer review effectively as well as on their ability to write successfully. The peer-review rubric is taught in class using multiple examples from previous classes, such as the two quoted earlier in this article. In peer reviewing another student's work, students derive several benefits besides editorial assistance. They are able to "meet," at least on paper, several volunteers besides their own. They are exposed to different ways of organizing and presenting similar data, and they are able to view another future clinician's clinical reasoning as they begin to develop their own skills in critical thinking (Bean, 1996).

Students are also asked to attend three meetings of a community support group for people with disabilities and to report verbally on these meetings to the class. In this way, students become aware of the kinds of peer counseling and coaching (Vash, 1981) and community support available to people with disabilities outside of the family and the health care system. Some support groups ask the students to do a presentation to the group, benefiting both the student and the group. As the Internet becomes a more popular form of communication for those who lack mobility or facile speech, some online support groups have been added to the array of students' local support group opportunities.

Evaluations of the course by students and evaluation of the students by volunteers both show positive outcomes in the students' ability to establish meaningful and comfortable relationships with people with disabilities and to recognize the impact of disability on human occupation. The volunteers report that they enjoy the opportunity to educate budding young health professionals on the topic of living with a disability. The students report an appreciation of the meaning of disability to the person who is disabled, in a naturalistic setting (Moyers, 1999). Typical comments from student evaluations of the course include:

This course contained more self-learning than in other courses where we learned out of a book. I learned about interviewing, evaluating, and disability in general.

The interactions with our volunteers were extremely helpful in that they provided insight into another person's perspective.

The assignment that benefited me the most was the community outing. This is the time where I learned the most about my volunteer and the way she functions with her disability.

The assessments on accessibility in the home and community gave me a good understanding of the challenges facing someone in a wheelchair.

The volunteers, when asked to rate the performance of their students, reported the following:

Although I was experiencing great cognitive and emotional problems, stress over recent job loss, etc., Nancy jumped right in with me and worked at my pace with great caring and understanding. . . . Nancy did something no other student I've had has done; she inquired about my ideas as to how there could be correlations between mental illness and O.T. services.

His non-assuming approach provides an openness that allows for the development of communication, which is essential in being effective toward helping others to reach their goals. His demonstration of his willingness to learn and participate in his clients' unfolding of their own understanding of what they have to deal with is especially comforting. These key essentials which are necessary for being a good therapist are traits which he has demonstrated in a very real way.

In summary, *Disability in Context* expands placement opportunities while offering a positive and viable fieldwork experience with people who have disabling conditions. It integrates didactic with experiential learning regarding human occupation, using a cooperative teaching model (Johnson, Johnson, & Smith, 1991). It promotes a mutual exchange in teaching/learning between volunteer and student and allows the volunteer to offer students a view of disability from the perspective of someone who actually lives with a disabling condition. As practice shifts toward being consumer-driven and community-based, courses such as this one offer students an appreciation of people with disabilities being in charge of their own lives, and help students view disability within the context of a lived experience.

REFERENCES

Accreditation Council for Occupational Therapy Education. (1998). Standards for an accredited educational program for the occupational therapist. *American Journal of Occupational Therapy, 53* (6), 575-582.

Barnes, M.A., & Evenson, M.E. (2000). Lesson 6: Meeting the fieldwork challenge. Structuring learning experiences. In S.C. Merrill & P. Crist (Eds.), *Meeting the fieldwork challenge: A self-paced clinical course from AOTA* (Lessons 1-11). Bethesda, MD: American Occupational Therapy Association.

Bean, J.C. (1996). *Engaging ideas.* San Francisco: Jossey-Bass.

Borcherding, S. (2000). *A documentation manual for writing SOAP notes in occupational therapy.* Thorofare, NJ: Slack.

Bowen, R.E. (1996). The issue is: Should occupational therapy adopt a consumer-based model of service delivery? *American Journal of Occupational Therapy, 50* (10), 899-902.

Davis, C. (1998). *Patient practitioner interaction.* Thorofare, NJ: Slack.

Department of Occupational Therapy. (1998). *Department of Occupational Therapy philosophy* (revised). Columbia: University of Missouri-Columbia.

Fazio, L.S. (2001). *Developing occupation-centered programs for the community: A workbook for students and professionals.* Upper Saddle River, NJ: Prentice Hall.

Johnson, D.W., Johnson, R.T., & Smith, K.A. (1991). *Cooperative learning: Increasing college faculty instructional productivity* (ASHE-ERIC Higher Education Report no. 4). Washington, DC: George Washington University.

Kielhofner, G. (1995). *A model of human occupation: Theory and application.* Baltimore: Williams & Wilkins.

Law, M. (1998). *Client-centered occupational therapy.* Thorofare, NJ: Slack.

McColl, M.A., Gerein, N., & Valentine, F. (1997). Meeting the challenges of disability: Models for enabling function and well-being. In C. Christiansen & C. Baum (Eds.), *Occupational therapy: Enabling function and well-being* (2nd ed., pp. 508-528). Thorofare, NJ: Slack.

Moyers, P.A. (1999). The guide to occupational therapy practice. *American Journal of Occupational Therapy [Special issue],* 53(3).

Oakley, F. (1982). *The model of human occupation in psychiatry.* Unpublished master's thesis, Virginia Commonwealth University, Richmond.

PEW Health Professions Commission. (1992). *Summary. Healthy America: Practitioners for 2005. A beginning dialogue for U.S. schools of allied health.* San Francisco: Center for the Health Professions, University of California.

Rydeen, K., Kautzmann, L., Cowan, M.K., & Benzing, P. (1995). Three faculty-facilitated, community-based level I fieldwork programs. *American Journal of Occupational Therapy, 49* (2), 112-118.

Smart, J. (2001). *Disability, society, and the individual.* Gaithersburg, MD: Aspen.

Smith, R.S., Kielhofner, G., & Watts, J.H. (1986). The relationships between volition, activity pattern, and life satisfaction in the elderly. *American Journal of Occupational Therapy, 40* (4), 278-283.

Trombly, C.A., & Versluys, H.P. (1989). Environmental evaluation and community reintegration. In C.A. Trombly (Ed.), *Occupational therapy for physical dysfunction* (3rd ed., pp. 427-440). Baltimore: Williams & Wilkins.

Vash, C.L. (1981). Volume 1: The psychology of disability. In T.B. Backer (Ed.), *Springer series on rehabilitation* (Vols. 1-3). New York: Springer.

World Health Organization. ICIDH-2: International classification of functioning, disability and health. Prefinal draft full version December 2000. World Health Organization home page. Retrieved February 15, 2001 from the World Wide Web: *http://www.who.icidh/ICIDH-2PFDec-2000.pdf*

Using Instructional Games:
A Teaching Strategy for Increasing
Student Participation and Retention

Kathy E. Gifford, MA, OTR/L

SUMMARY. Teaching occupational therapy intervention with sexual expression issues in the physically disabled population can be a challenging matter. Students are often uncomfortable with the subject matter, and this deters asking questions and becoming involved in the content to the extent of understanding the subject. Standard classroom approaches can be an ineffective match for teaching subjects requiring self-examination of attitudes. Rather than utilizing standard lecture or audiovisual techniques to engage students in knowledge transfer, this article describes an innovative game designed to help students explore their views on sexuality and learn about issues related to sexual expression for persons with physical disabilities. The rationale for such an activity is presented, as well as an overview of the game, rules, and procedures. Sample game items are included to give the reader a clearer idea of the game's content and focus. Student responses to the game are included. *[Article copies available for a fee from The Haworth Document Delivery Service: 1-800-HAWORTH. E-mail address: <getinfo@haworthpressinc. com> Website: <http://www.HaworthPress.com> © 2001 by The Haworth Press, Inc. All rights reserved.]*

Kathy E. Gifford is Assistant Professor, University of South Alabama, Department of Occupational Therapy, Mobile, AL.

[Haworth co-indexing entry note]: "Using Instructional Games: A Teaching Strategy for Increasing Student Participation and Retention." Gifford, Kathy E. Co-published simultaneously in *Occupational Therapy in Health Care* (The Haworth Press, Inc.) Vol. 15, No. 1/2, 2001, pp. 13-21; and: *Education for Occupational Therapy in Health Care: Strategies for the New Millennium* (eds: Patricia Crist, and Marjorie Scaffa) The Haworth Press, Inc., 2001, pp. 13-21. Single or multiple copies of this article are available for a fee from The Haworth Document Delivery Service [1-800-HAWORTH, 9:00 a.m. - 5:00 p.m. (EST). E-mail address: getinfo@haworthpressinc.com].

13

KEYWORDS. Educational games, innovative teaching, sexual expression

I hear and I forget
I see and I remember
Involve me and I understand

–Confucius

INTRODUCTION

Traditional classroom methods for teaching are predicated on the theory of knowledge transfer. Lecture and print-based audiovisual media are designed on the basis of this approach to learning. This theoretical approach assumes:

- A teacher is a necessary component for learning to take place
- The teacher is the source of knowledge
- The teacher organizes and transmits the knowledge to the students
- Knowledge transfer occurs in the classroom setting
- Learning has taken place when the message received is equivalent to the message sent. (Rubin, 1999)

Knowledge transfer theory does not allow for performance-based learning or development of appropriate attitudes that prepare the student for the work environment they will experience as an occupational therapist.

Today's student must be able to assimilate information into meaningful patterns of behavior. This is the desired outcome or end product of the educational process. To accomplish this they construct their own knowledge base from experiences both inside and outside the classroom. What the student knows must be used to determine "right actions." Conversely, knowledge transfer works best when the situation is almost, if not identical, to the one in which the content was presented (Ormrod, 1995). The knowledge transfer theory has little capacity to accommodate issues of linking knowledge with practice or emotions. Educators need tools for creating a learning environment that is rich in contextual elements to better prepare students for their roles as practitioners.

Gaming as an instructional tool is typically used for its concreteness: its ability to present abstract concepts in a way that requires the learner to be active in the process of grasping the content. Classroom games and simulations:

- Require application of knowledge with a context
- Can motivate learners

- Are fun
- Allow practice of skills

Research has shown instructors who integrate elements of play such as gaming into their teaching approach find students retain more knowledge and enjoy the learning more (Boettcher, Hahn, & Shaw, 1994).

Generally, for a skill to be mastered the learner must practice multiple times and be required to integrate the behavior in a variety of settings. Role play can be a helpful tool to beginning this process of skill development where the student is practicing how to interact with the patient, including using appropriate terminology and overcoming his/her fears or discomfort in dealing with issues a patient may present. During a game the student may experience some situations commonly encountered by practitioners and begin to apply information and practice professional communication skills. An instructional game can provide a more realistic context for applying and practicing skills without the consequences that are normally part of the therapist-patient interaction. Additionally, students can be asked to examine their attitudes and beliefs as a preparatory activity for patient interaction. Opportunities exist in a game situation to apply or determine "right actions" in a less threatening environment.

Occupational therapy students are trained to use concepts of adaptation to intervene when patients are experiencing or are at risk for problems in the area of sexual expression. This is a sensitive subject to effectively teach. Embarrassment frequently prevents students from asking questions or contributing to class discussion. Ultimately, students must become comfortable with applying the knowledge they have about sexual expression problems and adaptation concepts to real situations. Embarrassment and fear factors often interfere with reaching this level of learning. Therefore, alternatives for instruction are needed. Below is a description of "The Sex & Disability Game," an original game designed for use in teaching this content. It has been used multiple times to teach a unit on sexual expression instead of more traditional lectures or audiovisual formats of instruction. The unit is part of a course titled "Assessment & Therapy II" that is focused on the occupational therapy process applied to the adult population with physical disabilities.

Revisions have been made to the content and process based upon student feedback gathered at the conclusion of the game. Although the game was designed with occupational therapy students in mind, it has potential to be used in other settings where health care professionals need training to deal with sexuality and sexual expression issues of their clients.

STUDENTS

The students who are playing this game are in their junior year of the occupational therapy program. In addition to taking the above-mentioned course in assessment and therapy skills, they are enrolled in a course that addresses the dynamics of interpersonal relationships including a focus on appropriate professional communication skills and attitudes. They are also completing their first Fieldwork I in pediatrics. They will complete their Fieldwork Level I in adult physical disabilities settings in the following semester. The following is a description of the game and samples of game cards.

PURPOSE

The purpose of the game is to:

1. Have the students explore their attitudes about their sexuality and the sexuality of persons with disabilities.
2. Expand their knowledge of how disability affects sexual expression.
3. Develop their knowledge of adaptations appropriate to compensating for difficulties in sexual functioning due to a physical disability.
4. Develop the students' skill in handling common situations concerning sexuality which arise with patients in clinical practice.

LEARNING OBJECTIVES

After playing the "Sex & Disability Game" for 45 minutes the students will:

1. Demonstrate awareness of their personal attitudes towards sexual expression.
2. Express increased comfort with open discussion of sexuality and sexual expression.
3. Define an appropriate role for the occupational therapist in intervention with persons experiencing problems with sexual expression. Be able to discern problem areas in sexual expression that are outside the scope of OT practice which, therefore, require referral to other professionals for assistance.
4. Possess knowledge of how physical disabilities can impede self-esteem, self-concept, and sexual expression.
5. Apply a variety of adaptation strategies to a patient-specific problem in sexual expression.

ORGANIZATION OF THE GAME

The game is non-competitive, meaning there are no winners or losers. The students are divided into small groups. The number of students per group can vary from 5 to10. Smaller numbers require more frequent responses from each member. Larger groups demand a higher trust level among group members. The students should be positioned in a circle facing center with no barriers, such as desks or tables, in front of them.

TOOLS

The game tools are stacks of five color-coded cards (blue, orange, green, yellow, pink) and a single die to roll to determine what type of card the player must draw. No answers are provided on the cards. The students must reference their textbooks for the answers if needed. The cards are color coded by topic:

Attitude Cards (blue). Questions on these cards are designed to explore personal attitudes about sexuality, as this is part of becoming comfortable in helping patients deal with sexual issues. Some cards in this category also ask questions pertaining to the student's attitude toward sexual expression in persons who are elderly and/or disabled.

Example Attitude Card:
"Do you consider flirting a compliment or an insult? If a patient flirts with you, how do you interpret the gesture?"

Sex and Adaptation Card (orange). Questions on these cards are designed to allow the students to discuss in a small group, appropriate suggestions or information to give to patients who are experiencing specific sexual functioning problems related to their disability. The students have assigned readings about adaptation to physical disability that they are expected to complete before class the day the game is played. Additionally, to prepare them for the game, students are instructed to utilize the professional communication skills learned in another course they are taking concurrently. This course addresses the need for respect for differences in individuals and the patients' right to autonomy and dignity.

Example Sex and Adaptation Card:
"If a patient has leg spasms frequently, name one adaptation you would suggest to him/her to manage the problem during sexual activity."

Sex and Disability Cards (green). These cards are designed to check the students' understanding of how various physical disabilities affect sexual functioning.

Example Sex and Disability Card:
"Are males with spinal cord injuries still fertile?"

Role Play Card (pink). When students select a role play card they are given a situation where they must play the part of an occupational therapist while the student seated next to them plays the role of a patient, and they act out the situation with the peer. Following each role play, all players are allowed to give their input about the situation.

Example Role Play Card:
"During ADL retraining with a male patient, he gets an erection. How do you respond?"

Pass Card (yellow). All players get one yellow card that they retain until they draw a question where they would like to defer their response. They may only defer a response to the game question once throughout the entire game. When they are turning in their yellow pass card, the play goes on to the next person who rolls the die for a new question.

Note–In the history of using this teaching tool none of the students in the last class used their "Pass Card." However, when the instructor asked about their opinion of the "Pass Card," the students reported that having it as part of the game was important to their comfort playing the game. The uncertainty they felt in playing a game focused on a sensitive subject was somewhat relieved by knowing they could use the "Pass Card" if needed. They felt it was an option should the question or situation on the card they drew be out of their comfort zone for discussing with the group.

DEBRIEFING

One of the key elements distinguishing play strictly carried out for enjoyment from games used for educational purposes is the need for debriefing. For the instructor, this portion of the process is the most challenging to do. Fuszard (1995) states that the instructor's task is to make the connection for the student between the game and reality. The game concept imparts a playfulness that contrasts with the seriousness of the topic. Dealing with sexual functioning and sexual expression problems in persons with new and/or permanent disabilities requires tact, utmost respect, and empathy for the patient. There is a strong demand to preserve human dignity throughout all aspects of the intervention. Reflection is necessary for students to return from the light-hearted play atmosphere created by the game to the seriousness of their role in helping patients cope with sexual expression issues. During this time, the instructor has the opportunity to connect the process of the game (a fictitious situation) with real-life situations a therapist may face in the clinic. Opportunities for reflection beyond simply debriefing are a necessary component to make this connection.

Student reflection should include an awareness of crucial issues, should involve respect for the patient, and should duly deal with the needs of the patient in a responsible manner. This can be done in a written format. Students who have played this game in class have been asked to write about the experience.

First the students are involved in a debriefing where they have an opportunity to ask any questions that may have come up during the game. They are asked to reflect on their responses to the game both collectively, as group members, and individually and what they learned. They are required to write about the benefits and suggestions they have to improve the game. Students reported increased personal comfort with the topic and most felt it was a fun way to learn about the topic. Their reflections included comments about how the game was a vehicle for reflection about their attitudes, values and beliefs about sexuality. They often commented on how important it is to become more comfortable with the topic and be aware of situations that commonly occur in clinical settings. The instructor's role during this process is to facilitate the student's understanding of how to respond to patients' concerns with an attitude of openness, sincerity and understanding for the sensitive nature of the problem.

FEEDBACK

The following are some anonymous comments given by students following the game.

Positive

- Provides an opportunity to explore a serious and sometimes embarrassing subject in a nonthreatening environment
- Required us to read aloud embarrassing topics and address them in a mature way
- Having the Pass Card eased anxiety, even though no one used it
- Required thinking and problem solving
- The scenarios required thinking about situations that may happen in the "real world"

- Role play required a way to practice what to say and how to say it
- Increased comfort discussing the topic amongst peers in small groups instead of as a class.

Negative

- People just agreed with others' responses to "Attitude cards" rather than thinking of their own response
- No answer key to the non-opinion type questions for corrective feedback
- Some questions were so vague, they were difficult to interpret
- Role play is difficult because the other party is a peer
- It is hard to role play some scenarios because they are serious in nature but the atmosphere of game playing made everyone more light-hearted.

Additionally, during the debriefing, the students have been asked to develop a question that they feel could be added to the game. Some of their questions have been added. Some were revised for clarification and then added to the game to make a few new questions each year. Some questions submitted were not congruent with the scope and objectives of the game. Students worked with the instructor to improve the question format for inclusion into the game. By having them think of questions, they again were required to review the content already covered in the existing questions, and add relevant new questions on the topic.

CONCLUSION

Classroom teaching should include a variety of learning strategies to create interest in students and address differences in learning styles. Knowledge transfer does not work best for some situations. Students need learning experiences that require active participation and synthesis of content to prepare them for clinical practice. Creativeness is also an essential ability of an effective occupational therapist. Opportunities to "think and apply information outside the box" facilitate problem solving and innovativeness in students. Exploring the self and one's own views of sexuality help reveal areas where students may feel uncomfortable and which need to be resolved before moving into the clinical setting. Respect for human dignity and sensitivity are paramount in the subject area of sexual expression. The instructor can provide or reinforce this issue during the debriefing of the game.

Gaming can be an effective approach to instruction when the desired outcomes are: a change in attitude, increased ability to problem solve, or creative approaches to practical situations. Students usually love the change of pace. It piques their interest. Study of neuroscience indicates that we remember best those events that are associated with strong emotions, which, of course, include enjoyment (Guyton, 1991).

REFERENCES

Boettcher, W.S., Hahn, S.S., & Shaw, G.L. (1994). Mathematics and music: A search for insight into higher brain function. *Leonardo Music Journal, 4*, 53-58.

Fuszard, B. (1995). *Innovative Teaching Strategies in Nursing* (2nd ed.), p. 116. Gaithersburg, MD: Aspen Publications, Inc.

Guyton, A. (1991). The cerebral cortex: Intellectual functions of the brain and learning and memory. In *Basic Neuroscience* (2nd ed.), Philadelphia: W. B. Saunders, p. 252.

Ormrod, J. (1995). Transfer and problem solving. In *Human Learning*, Edgewood Cliffs, NJ: Prentice-Hall, Inc., pp. 371-372.

Ruben, B. (Dec., 1999). Simulations, games and experience-based learning: The quest for a new paradigm for teaching and learning. *Simulation & Gaming, 30* (4), 498.

The Fieldwork Profile:
A Statistics Assignment Linked
to the Real World
of Occupational Therapy Students

Marcia Finlayson, PhD, OT (C), OTR/L

SUMMARY. New accreditation standards state that an entry-level occupational therapist who graduates from an accredited program should be an effective research consumer and should possess basic skills as a researcher. Some of these basic skills include being able to organize, collect, and analyze data to evaluate practice outcomes and being able to understand, use, and interpret statistics, specifically those which are descriptive, correlational, and inferential. Facilitating the development of these skills requires innovative and meaningful research assignments during occupational therapy education. The purpose of this article is to describe an applied statistics assignment based on the premise of learning-by-doing. The assignment is known as the "fieldwork profile analysis" and provides students an opportunity to connect their fieldwork experiences to their research class. Students responded posi-

Marcia Finlayson is Assistant Professor, Department of Occupational Therapy (MC 811), University of Illinois at Chicago, 1919 West Taylor Street, Chicago, IL 60612 (E-mail: marciaf@uic.edu).

This assignment was used by Dr. Finlayson during her employment at Nova Southeastern University in Ft. Lauderdale, FL.

[Haworth co-indexing entry note]: "The Fieldwork Profile: A Statistics Assignment Linked to the Real World of Occupational Therapy Students." Finlayson, Marcia. Co-published simultaneously in *Occupational Therapy in Health Care* (The Haworth Press, Inc.) Vol. 15, No. 1/2, 2001, pp. 23-30; and: *Education for Occupational Therapy in Health Care: Strategies for the New Millennium* (eds: Patricia Crist, and Marjorie Scaffa) The Haworth Press, Inc., 2001, pp. 23-30. Single or multiple copies of this article are available for a fee from The Haworth Document Delivery Service [1-800-HAWORTH, 9:00 a.m. - 5:00 p.m. (EST). E-mail address: getinfo@haworthpressinc.com].

23

tively to the assignment and indicated that their active involvement doing statistics facilitated their learning. *[Article copies available for a fee from The Haworth Document Delivery Service: 1-800-HAWORTH. E-mail address: <getinfo@haworthpressinc.com> Website: <http://www.HaworthPress. com> © 2001 by The Haworth Press, Inc. All rights reserved.]*

KEYWORDS. Graduate education, statistics, learning-by-doing

In April 1999, the Representative Assembly of the American Occupational Therapy Association adopted Resolution J supporting a post-baccalaureate degree in occupational therapy as the required level of education for entry into the profession (Steib, 1999). Regardless of discipline, a masters level education implies an advanced level of knowledge in a particular area of study. In many fields, it also implies that the graduate has knowledge and skills in research design and analysis. The new accreditation standards for occupational therapist educational programs, effective July 2000, identify research skills and knowledge as critical for the entry level occupational therapist (Accreditation Council for Occupational Therapy Education [ACOTE], 1999). Being able to understand, use, and interpret descriptive, correlational, and inferential statistics are just three of the specific research related skills identified in the new standards.

Research and statistics are not typically the favorite classes in an occupational therapy program, as they often do not connect to the real world of the student. Other disciplines and fields also have this problem (Yilmaz, 1996). While some students approach research and statistics classes with curiosity, many more students are tentative about what lies ahead and carry attitudes and fears that can hamper their ability to learn statistics (Hogg, 1991). The challenge faced by the research professor is not only to overcome this tentativeness but to instill in students an appreciation and excitement for the possibilities of research, a realization that research and statistics are relevant to their future professional practice, and a desire to be involved in some way in the research process after graduation.

Encouraging and facilitating future involvement in research requires innovative and meaningful research assignments during occupational therapy education that will stay with students and provide ideas and templates for research in their future. Developing assignments with these characteristics requires occupational therapy educators to operationalize one of the most basic premises of occupational therapy: learning-by-doing.

The purpose of this article is to describe an applied statistics assignment based on this premise. The assignment is known as the "fieldwork profile analysis" and was given to second-year students in a post-baccalaureate entry-level occupational therapy program at one private university during the 1998-99 and 1999-2000 academic years.

ASSIGNMENT CONTEXT

The "fieldwork profile analysis" is an assignment in the second of two research methods courses that are required in the second year of a 30-month post-baccalaureate entry-level program. The first course focuses on foundation content. Students learn about worldviews and paradigms and their influence on research, ways of identifying research topics, as well as about searching the literature, developing questions, choosing methodologies and methods, sampling, and applying ethical principles. The second research course moves on to the details of planning a study, preparing an Institutional Review Board submission, and learning statistical as well as qualitative analysis.

During the first half of the second research methods course, students take a six-week section on statistics that includes both didactic classes and computer labs. Students are introduced to measures of central tendency, measures of variability, the normal distribution (as well as the t-test), one-way analysis of variance, correlations, and the chi-squared test. During the computer labs, students have the opportunity to apply what they have learned in the didactic classes. Throughout the statistics sessions, emphasis is placed on the theory behind the tests and problem-solving rather than on memorizing formulas. This focus is consistent with that advocated by Hogg (1991) and others. Students are expected to be able to explain what the test does, what types of variables (e.g., interval, nominal, binomial) are needed to run the test, and the assumptions of the tests (e.g., normal distribution, homogeneity of variance). Students are also taught how to ensure that test assumptions are met and what to do in case they are not. Students learn how to state null, non-directional, and directional hypotheses, determine whether they are accepted or rejected, and to explain what the findings mean.

THE ASSIGNMENT: THE FIELDWORK PROFILE

The Fieldwork Profile is an assignment that contains three basic components–data collection, data entry and management, and data analysis and dissemination. As a result, this assignment alone does not cover the entire research process or all of the skills identified in the ACOTE standards. Rather, the focus of the Fieldwork Profile Assignment is on learning statistics by actively completing a statistical analysis to answer a specific question. This approach is encouraged by authors such as Smith (1998) and Gnanadesikan, Scheaffer, Watkins, and Witmer (1997). The primary research question that guided this assignment was: What are the differences in the experiences of students completing different types of fieldwork? The rationale for the question was that students who were going to nontraditional fieldwork sites were expressing concern that they were not developing the same skills as their peers who were doing fieldwork in traditional sites. The fieldwork profile assignment allowed students to explore the accuracy of their own perceptions.

Part I: Data Collection—Completing the Fieldwork Data Sheets

The first part of the fieldwork profile involves data collection and is completed by students while they are on their Level I fieldwork rotations, which are three weeks in duration. Students record their fieldwork experiences on a data collection form provided to them, which has been approved by the University's Institutional Review Board (IRB). Each student collects information related to the student-client interaction and its context during fieldwork (e.g., sex and age of clients seen, the primary performance areas and components for intervention, the number of one-to-one and group contacts the student has with each client). In addition, the student records general information, such as the month of the placement, the type of supervision he/she received (OTR versus non-OTR), the type of setting (e.g., hospital, school), and the specific rotation being completed (e.g., older adults, mental health).

Upon returning to classes after fieldwork, students must show their completed data sheets to the professor. Students are instructed on proper storage of their data and are responsible for maintaining its security until the following semester.

Part II: Data Entry and Management

During the statistics section of the second research methods course, students work with the data they have collected. During the first statistics computer lab, students learn how to create a data set and enter their data. Students create identical data sets using their own data, following written instructions provided by the professor. Students are also instructed on how to use univariate analyses to check and clean their data to ensure that they have not made any data entry errors. Upon completion of data entry and cleaning, students submit their data sets to the professor, who merges all of the data into a single data set. Merging the data was not done during the first year of this assignment (1998-99). For some students, this resulted in small sample sizes and inadequate statistical power. During the 1999-2000 academic year, the data were merged, providing students with a data set with N = 3,816 clients. The merged data set was copied onto the students' disks and returned to them for analysis.

Part III: Data Analysis and Dissemination

The final part of the assignment requires students to analyze the merged field-work data set to answer the primary research question (i.e., What are the differences in the experiences of students completing different types of fieldwork?). Students are instructed on how to run and present descriptive statistics on the variables they have chosen to use for their tests. Each student must pose specific secondary research questions based on the primary question. Students must also set hypotheses for each one of the statistical tests that he/she must run: a t-test, an ANOVA, a correlation, and a chi-squared test. Examples of questions posed by students include: Is there a difference in the average age of clients seen in community versus medical settings? Is there a relationship between the age of the client and the number of group contacts occurring between students and clients?

Students are guided through the process of confirming the assumptions of each test and of how to problem-solve when a test's assumptions are not met. They are also provided instruction and reference materials on how to write up their findings using appropriate language (Lang & Secic, 1997). The capstone of the student's work is a paper that must include an introduction, a method description, an explanation of the results, and an overall conclusion.

DOES THE ASSIGNMENT WORK?

While no formal evaluation of the fieldwork profile assignment has been completed, students did provide written feedback on all of the research methods assignments in both the 1998-99 and 1999-2000 academic years. Students completed a total of seven major assignments in the research methods courses. In addition to the fieldwork profile, students completed a series of linked assignments that took them through the entire research process, including preparing a study rationale, completing a literature search, writing a literature review, choosing a design and method, preparing an IRB submission, and completing and analysing two qualitative interviews. Considering all but the last assignment, since it had not yet been completed at the time feedback was provided, students were asked: (1) Which assignment was the most intellectually challenging for you? (2) Which assignment gave you the greatest appreciation for the complexity of research? (3) From which assignments did you learn the most for the time you spent on them?

The responses of the 152 students (response rate = 99%) are summarized in Table 1. Examples of their qualitative comments relating to the fieldwork profile included:

The fieldwork profile analysis was the most intellectually challenging because it forced me to truly understand the material and apply what I had learned.

The fieldwork profile analysis was the most challenging because I had never done anything like that before. I had to learn all new info on SPSS and all four tests. Then I had to write a paper on the findings. It took a lot of problem solving and critical thinking to figure it out.

The fieldwork profile analysis assignment [was the most challenging] because I struggle with trying to understand statistics. The primary focus of my former stats class was plugging numbers into formulas, but the meaning of the results were not clearly explained. This assignment forced me to understand what I was doing and WHY!

The fieldwork profile [gave me the greatest appreciation] because I learned how hard it is to read tests and understand the findings. It was amazing to me that in research the memorizing doesn't do you any good. You really have to understand and apply the information.

I learned the most from the profile analysis because I had the chance to try to apply the knowledge as soon as I could understand a concept. It took a while, but it turned out to be the most meaningful way for me to learn.

While the comments above do not indicate the effectiveness of the Fieldwork Profile assignment, they do support the notion that engagement in the activity of statistical analysis was both intellectually challenging as well as academically rewarding for the students. Creating positive attitudes towards statistics and research in current occupational therapy students is critical for the future development of the profession.

CONCLUSION

Occupational therapists emphasize learning-by-doing and encouraging occupational engagement through the facilitation of meaningful activities. Occupational therapy educators must emphasize these same principles, regardless of the content area they are responsible for within a curriculum. The Fieldwork Profile assignment provides the opportunity to apply occupational therapy principles to the teaching of statistics while at the same time addressing *some* of the research skills addressed in the new ACOTE standards.

TABLE 1. Summary of Student Feedback on Research Assignments

Question	Number (%) of responses N = 152
Which assignment was the most intellectually challenging for you?	
Fieldwork profile	70 (46.1%)
Rationale	6 (3.9%)
Literature search	4 (2.6%)
Critical literature review	51 (33.6%)
Choosing a design & method	14 (9.2%)
IRB submission	4 (2.6%)
Other	3 (2.0%)
Which assignment gave you the greatest appreciation for the complexity of research?	
Fieldwork profile	31 (20.4%)
Rationale	3 (2.0%)
Literature search	5 (3.3%)
Critical literature review	25 (16.4%)
Choosing a design & method	12 (7.9%)
IRB submission	52 (34.2%)
Other	24 (15.8%)
From which assignments did you learn the most for the time you spent on them?*	
Response includes fieldwork profile	112 (73.7%)
Response does not include fieldwork profile	20 (26.3%)

*Students could identify up to two assignments when answering this question, and, therefore, the descriptive analysis coded responses as including or not including the fieldwork profile.

Through this assignment, students develop basic skills of organizing, collecting and analyzing data, and understanding, using, and interpreting statistics. The assignment also provides students with the opportunity to develop basic skills necessary for publication and presentation of research activities. Further development of the fieldwork profile holds the possibility of being able to address the entire research process within this assignment. Since fieldwork is such an important and meaningful component of occupational therapy education, linking the experience of fieldwork to a statistics assignment helped make statistics "real" for students.

There is very little literature available on teaching statistics to occupational therapy students, but periodicals such as the *Journal of Statistics Education* and the *American Statistician* are great resources for educators in the position of having to teach this material. Learning statistics by doing statistics offers students the opportunity to engage in active learning (Gnanadesikan et al., 1997) to develop "skills such as the ability to interpret, evaluate and apply statistical ideas" (Chance, 1997, p. 1), to practice statistical reasoning and problem-solving (Chance, 1997), and to learn to write and present statistical findings (Smith, 1998).

REFERENCES

Accreditation Council for Occupational Therapy Education (ACOTE). (1999). *Standards for an accredited educational program for the occupational therapist.* Bethesda, MD: AOTA, Inc. Full text available on-line at: *http://www.aota.org/nonmembers/area9/links/LINK03.asp*

Chance, B.L. (1997). Experiences with authentic assessment techniques in an introductory statistics course. *Journal of Statistics Education, 5* (3). Full text available on-line at: *http://www.amstat.org/publications/jse/v5n3/chance.html*

Gnanadesikan, M., Scheaffer, R.L., Watkins, A.E., & Witmer, J.A. (1997). An activity-based statistics course. *Journal of Statistics Education, 5* (2). Full text available on-line at: *http://www.amstat.org/publications/jse/v5n2/gnanadesikan.html*

Hogg, R.V. (1991). Statistical education: Improvements are badly needed. *The American Statistician, 45,* 342-343.

Lang, T.A., & Secic, M. (1997). *How to report statistics in medicine: Annotated guidelines for authors, editors and reviewers.* Philadelphia, PA: American College of Physicians.

Smith, G. (1998). Learning statistics by doing statistics. *Journal of Statistics Education, 6* (3). Full text available on-line at: *http://www.amstat.org/publications/jse/v6n3/smith.html*

Steib, P. (1999). 1999 RA makes history: Resolution J adopted. *OT Week, 13* (16), i & iii.

Yilmaz, M.R. (1996). The challenge of teaching statistics to non-specialists. *Journal of Statistics Education, 4* (1). Full text available on-line at: *http://www.amstat.org/publications/jse/v4n1/yilmaz.html*

Understanding Others:
A Course to Learn
Interactive Clinical Reasoning

Diana M. Bailey, EdD, OTR/L, FAOTA
Ellen S. Cohn, ScD, OTR/L, FAOTA

SUMMARY. Teaching future practitioners to use clinical reasoning processes is necessary for entry-level practice. While there are numerous articles addressing some aspects of clinical reasoning, none describe a course solely focused on understanding another person's perspective–interactive clinical reasoning. The article describes an Interactive Clinical Reasoning course for entry-level graduate students–one of four seminars on clinical reasoning embedded in a curriculum that simultaneously uses an infusion model to increase cultural awareness and sensitivity.

Diana M. Bailey is Associate Professor, Tufts University- Boston School of Occupational Therapy, Medford, MA 02115. She has co-taught the Interactive Clinical Reasoning course with Dr. Cohn on many occasions, in addition to several other courses in clinical reasoning. Her publications have centered around research methods, health care policy, and management issues–courses she teaches at Tufts University.

Ellen S. Cohn is Clinical Associate Professor, Boston University, Sargent College, Department of Occupational Therapy, Boston, MA. She was formerly a faculty member at Tufts University-Boston School of Occupational Therapy where she co-taught clinical reasoning courses with Dr. Bailey. Dr. Cohn was a member of the AOTA/AOTF Clinical Reasoning Research Team and has published extensively in the area of clinical reasoning and fieldwork education.

Address correspondence to: Dr. Ellen Cohn, Boston University, Sargent College, Department of Occupational Therapy, 635 Commonwealth Avenue, SAR551, Boston, MA 02215 (E-mail: ecohn@bu.edu).

[Haworth co-indexing entry note]: "Understanding Others: A Course to Learn Interactive Clinical Reasoning." Bailey, Diana M., and Ellen S. Cohn. Co-published simultaneously in *Occupational Therapy in Health Care* (The Haworth Press, Inc.) Vol. 15, No. 1/2, 2001, pp. 31-46; and: *Education for Occupational Therapy in Health Care: Strategies for the New Millennium* (eds: Patricia Crist, and Marjorie Scaffa) The Haworth Press, Inc., 2001, pp. 31-46. Single or multiple copies of this article are available for a fee from The Haworth Document Delivery Service [1-800-HAWORTH, 9:00 a.m. - 5:00 p.m. (EST). E-mail address: getinfo@haworthpressinc.com].

31

The underlying philosophy of the course includes using interpersonal intelligence (Gardner, 1985) to "treat a patient's illness experience" (Mattingly, 1992, p. 4). Clients are the experts of their own experience with illness or disability, and students must pay as much attention to their questions and their own reactions as to their interviewee's responses. Readings, videotapes, assignments, and class exercises designed to increase students' interviewing skills and their ability to understand each client's perspective are described. *[Article copies available for a fee from The Haworth Document Delivery Service: 1-800-HAWORTH. E-mail address: <getinfo@haworthpressinc.com> Website: <http://www.HaworthPress.com> © 2001 by The Haworth Press, Inc. All rights reserved.]*

KEYWORDS. Phenomenology, illness experience, cultural sensitivity

The occupational therapy literature is replete with calls to teach future practitioners the clinical reasoning processes necessary for entry-level practice (Cohn, 1989; Cohn, 1991; Mattingly & Fleming, 1994; Neistadt, 1987, 1992, 1996; Neistadt, Wight, & Mulligan, 1998; Parham, 1987; Rogers, 1983; Schell, 1998; Schell & Cervero, 1993; Schwartz, 1991). Educators are challenged to develop creative approaches to teaching because clinical reasoning involves more than a straightforward application of theory to practical problems. Clinical reasoning involves making judgments that are specific to a context, about how to provide intervention for a particular person, in a particular place and time. Occupational therapy is what occupational therapists do, and clinical reasoning is the process therapists use to frame problems, make sense of where they can go with particular clients, and decide what to do in the midst of practice. Clinical reasoning is a complex thinking process that happens over time; it is an interactive and unfolding process over the entire course of therapy. The purpose of this article is to describe a course taught within an occupational therapy curriculum that is based on a clinical reasoning framework. The course focuses on the interactive and phenomenological aspects of clinical reasoning.

In a comprehensive review of the occupational therapy clinical reasoning literature, Schell (1998) summarized four facets of clinical reasoning: scientific, pragmatic, ethical, and narrative reasoning. Based on Fleming's (1991) notion that therapists use multiple strands of reasoning, Schell reminds us that clinical reasoning is both an interactive and a conditional process. Together with their clients, occupational therapists co-construct a future story for the client, which they enact in the therapy process. In their efforts to engage clients in the therapy process, Mattingly (1991) proposed that therapists use a pheno-menological or interpretive approach to understanding how clients privately compose their experience of disease or disability and what brings meaning to their lives. Mattingly and Fleming (1994) have described the reasoning that guides this process as interactive reasoning. Thus we assume that therapists must strive to understand the client's perspective in order to co-construct an intervention that will genuinely address the client's desires.

TEACHING CLINICAL REASONING

Numerous authors in occupational therapy have described approaches for teaching aspects of clinical reasoning. In 1996, Neistadt reviewed the occupational therapy literature and categorized various approaches to teaching aspects of clinical reasoning. One teaching approach involves inviting guest speakers with various physical disabilities to role model as clients and simulate a practice environment to develop clinical reasoning skills in a problem-based learning format (Neistadt, 1987, 1992; Van Leit, 1995). To help students understand how different persons experience illness or disability, other authors have recommended reading and analyzing literature about disability experiences (Crepeau, 1991; Kautzmann, 1993; Peloquin, 1989, 1995), writing narratives about clients (Mattingly & Fleming, 1994), or writing autobiographical papers (Neistadt, 1996). Peloquin and Babola (1996) created a clinical climate in the classroom to help students make the transition between academic and clinical expectations and learn professional behavior. More recently, Neistadt, Wight, and Mulligan (1998) described a new type of written case study that models the clinical reasoning process by organizing client-related information according to the types of reasoning that would be used to gather that information. Neistadt (1998) also described a thinking-frame approach—an explicit structure to organize and support the thought processes necessary for clinical reasoning.

While all these teaching approaches address some aspect of clinical reasoning, none describes a course solely focused on preparing students to understand another person's perspective—interactive clinical reasoning. In her observations of the occupational therapy profession, Mattingly noted that there were no courses in occupational therapy curricula to "equip occupational therapy students to treat the phenomenological body" (Mattingly & Fleming, 1994, p. 75). Mattingly claims, "It is treating a patient's illness experience which is integral to good occupational therapy. This is where the heart of clinical reasoning lies, and where the thorniest reasoning puzzles present themselves. Reasoning about how to treat the illness experience is often the most difficult thing to teach" (1992, p. 4). Mattingly's observations highlight the importance of students learning how to relate to other people.

THE INTERACTIVE CLINICAL REASONING COURSE

The two-credit interactive reasoning course described in this article is situated in a 2.5-year curriculum designed for entry-level master's degree students. All students have a bachelor's degree in a field other than occupational therapy, and about two-thirds of them have been working in careers such as business, fine arts, or biology for 5 to 10 years prior to entering the program. Students' ages range from 22 years to 55 years, with the biggest cohort in their late 20s and early 30s. The course has been taught several times to class sizes ranging from 30 to 80 students; the small groups have varied from 5 to 10 students per group. Classes are held once per week in two-hour sessions, over a 12-13 week semester. Each class consists of a one-hour lecture and one hour for small group application of lecture or readings.

The interactive clinical reasoning course, taught during the spring semester of their first year, is part of a sequence of four courses aimed at systematically teaching students the conceptual and operational skills required to analyze clinical situations (Cohn, 1991). The first course on observation and interpretation addresses students' reasoning skills with an emphasis on the ability to make, reflect on, analyze, and critique observations and interpretations. The second course, focused on interactive reasoning, will be presented in detail in this article. In the third course, students examine the different procedures practitioners select when assessing and treating specific clients and the procedural or scientific reasoning behind their choices. The final course focuses on developing students' advanced analytical skills and a deeper understanding of the occupational therapists' role in the social reconstruction of the self.

Gardner (1985) proposed that there are several kinds of intelligence and that different results are achieved depending on the types of intelligence used. The interactive clinical reasoning course encourages students to use what Gardner refers to as "interpersonal intelligence" (p. 239). He postulates two types of interpersonal intelligence: "The capacity to access one's own feeling life" and "The ability to notice and make distinctions among other individuals, in particular among their moods, temperaments, motivations, and intentions" (p. 239). Gardner's ideas serve as the organizing framework for sequencing course materials and assignments. In a recursive manner, students are repeatedly analyzing their own feelings, values, and beliefs and using that analysis to inform their observations and interactions with others. Topics are ordered throughout the semester to allow students to achieve both knowledge and personal growth.

The course objectives are listed in Appendix A. The sequence of topics begins with an analysis of self (see Appendix B) in which students identify attributes about themselves in order to understand how these attributes influence their interactions. Throughout the semester, as students reflect on their interactions with others, they are encouraged to refer back to their analysis of self.

The clinical reasoning courses are part of a curriculum that uses an infusion model to teach cultural sensitivity, so that the importance of culture is emphasized throughout the students' program (Bailey, 2000). Thus, students in the interactive reasoning course already have a basic appreciation of major differences among people, such as race, ethnicity, religion, socioeconomic status, sexual orientation, disability, appearance, or age. To strengthen students' understanding of culture and phenomenology, lectures and videotapes addressing cultural sensitivity and language of disability are provided. In small groups, students engage in activities designed to increase their understanding of the influence of their own culture, family, development, and experiences with disability on the way they interact with others. (See Appendix C for an example of a small group activity designed to explore family values.) These activities culminate in an assignment in which students interview someone of their own choosing, from a culture other than their own.

To learn about interaction and the power of therapeutic relationships, students read selections from two required texts, *Clinical reasoning: Forms of inquiry in a therapeutic practice* (Mattingly & Fleming, 1994) and *Patient practitioner interaction: An experiential manual for developing the art of health care* (Davis, 1998). In addition, students are assigned other readings specific to the week's topic, such as sensitivity to the language of disability (Zola, 1993), empathy (Peloquin, 1995), white privilege (McIntosh, 1989), services for people with HIV/AIDS (AOTA, 1996), sensitivity to clients' sexual orientation (Jackson, 1995), the process of termination from the therapeutic relationship (Howe & Schwartzberg, 1995; Maholick & Turner, 1979; Martin & Berchule, 1988), and client empowerment (Emener, 1991).

Spencer, Krefting, and Mattingly (1993) advocate the use of qualitative methods, specifically ethnographic methods, to assess the meaning of occupation, the illness experience, and the context in which they occur. These authors explain that the object of ethnography is to understand another way of life from the participant's viewpoint within a cultural context and suggest that an ethnographic perspective yields a good understanding of ways to enhance engagement in occupation valued by the person. Using the ethnographic perspective advocated by Spencer and colleagues, the interactive reasoning course focuses on the interactive and phenomenological aspects of clinical reasoning in which students are taught a client-centered approach to interviewing people about their experiences living with a disease or disability.

Students practice asking specific questions and develop beginning interview techniques by conducting, analyzing, and videotaping an interview with a classmate at the beginning and again at the end of the course. Student interviewees complete portions of either the Role Check List (Barris, Oakley, & Kielhofner, 1988) or the Occupational Performance History Interview (Kielhofner, Henry, & Walens, 1989) in preparation for being interviewed. Using these occupational therapy tools helps students begin to think about roles and occupational themes in their own lives. Student interviewers analyze and evaluate their own videotapes for approaches used and the ability to establish rapport with the interviewee, to engage the interviewee in conversation, and to understand the interviewee's perspective. Students identify concerns, content, and affect they wish they had attended to and identify other approaches they might try if they had the opportunity to recreate the interview. The videotapes allow students to examine their word choice, intonation, rate of speech, body movements, and other nonverbal aspects of communication (Tickle-Degnen, 1995). By interviewing peers, students have the rare opportunity to receive direct feedback about their interviewing style as they process their interview and review the videotape with their classmate. Lectures and videotaped demonstrations of various interview concepts, such as opening an interview and asking open-ended, nonjudgmental questions, are provided early in the course. Small group exercises throughout the course give students the opportunity to practice: openings and endings for interviews, making topic transitions, setting limits and handling difficult moments, when and when not to self-disclose to a client, different types of body language, and designing and asking appropriate questions. Instructors occasionally role-play in small groups, and videotapes demonstrating specific points are discussed and techniques are tried out by students. A particularly valuable videotape is *Interviewing in action: Process and practice* (Murphy & Dillon, 1998). Once students have reflected on who they are and have practiced understanding their peers' perspectives, they prepare to interview guest speakers who are living with disabilities.

INTERVIEWING TO UNDERSTAND THE CLIENT'S PERSPECTIVE

A major premise of the course is that clients are the experts of their own experience with disability and the students' goal is to strive to understand the client's point of view and ways in which he/she constructs meaning in his/her life. Coles (1989) eloquently stated, "People who come to see us bring us their stories. They hope they will tell them well enough so that we understand the truth of their lives. They hope we will know how to interpret their stories correctly. We have to remember that it is their story" (p. 7).

In addition to Coles, we subscribe to Charmaz's view (1991), espoused when she was teaching interviewing skills to graduate sociology students:

> An interviewer must think continually about what this conversation seems to mean to the other person. Encouraging graduate students to do this helps them not only to understand the world view and experience of the people they happen to study but also to understand more clearly the role of language in explicating or obfuscating their world views and experience. (p. 388)

Only if practitioners listen to their clients' perceptions will they be able to join their clients in a collaborative partnership to design a successful intervention. In this course, students are invited to listen to guest speakers describe what life is like for them in their firsthand experience of living with disease or disability. Students are asked to listen to and interact with the guest speakers in order to understand the cultural context in which speakers live, the important people in their lives, what brings meaning to their lives, what they hope and dream for, and how they spend their time. Students prepare questions they will pose to a guest speaker; they hold a small-group interview with a guest speaker, then later analyze their questions and interview techniques in written assignments. Students' ability to listen is affected and influenced by who the students are themselves; therefore, we encourage them to use their analysis of self to understand as fully as possible the nature and extent of their own values and beliefs on their capacity to hear the speaker's story.

We invite guests living with HIV/AIDS, severe mental illness, mental retardation, spinal cord injury, and traumatic head injury to speak with small groups of students, followed by a group interview. Students are taught to view interviews as a dialogic process, a complex sequence of exchanges through which interviewer and interviewee negotiate some degree of agreement on what they will talk about and how (Mishler, 1986). This form of interviewing requires the interviewers (the students) to pay as much attention to the questions and their own reactions as to the interviewees' responses.

Students prepare for the interviews by investigating the speaker's disability and formulating a list of potential occupational performance problems with a rationale as to why that performance area might be impacted. This assignment encourages students to examine the judgments, or pre-interview hypotheses, they make based on a diagnosis and the limited information they know about their guest speaker prior to the interview. In addition to a diagnosis, other information includes gender, approximate age, living arrangements, and working status. Neistadt (1992) has advocated examining pre-judgments to teach students to revise their thinking and move beyond a diagnostic impression of a person. Based on their initial understanding of a particular diagnosis and the limited information they know about a guest speaker, students select five potential occupational performance problem areas and develop four questions about each occupation in order to gain a better understanding of what is important to that speaker. Each group of questions has a general opening question to introduce the topic to the guests, allowing the speakers to offer their own unique perspectives, and three follow-up questions addressing specific aspects of the performance area. During the interaction, students are expected to incorporate their knowledge of good interviewing questions (such as using open-ended, simple, positive, nonassumptive questions) and the interviewing techniques they have learned in the course (including body language, environmental setting, openings, transitions, and endings). Moreover, students often learn to be flexible and revise their interview questions in the midst of interactions as the guest speakers raise issues salient to their lives that students may not have considered in their pre-interview hypotheses.

There are three opportunities for students to meet with guests, and the expectation is that each interview will improve as students gain more experience. During processing sessions immediately following the interviews, students are encouraged to examine the presuppositions they held before meeting the speaker and their revised understanding and interpretation of the speaker's experience after the interview. Students strive to understand what life is like for the guest speaker and how their initial expectations may require reformulation based on a new understanding of a particular person in a particular context.

Rounding out the students' interviewing experience is a second videotaped peer interview at the end of the semester. Students compare their two interviews to examine their growth during the course; they look for improvement in their ability to engage and understand the interviewee, as well as in interviewing techniques. Students assess what more they need to learn or refine before they consider themselves competent interviewers from a phenomenological perspective.

EVALUATION OF THE INTERACTIVE CLINICAL REASONING COURSE

Course evaluations, completed anonymously by each student at the end of the interactive clinical reasoning course, tend to be favorable. Student comments reflect their growing awareness that knowing how to ask a question is as important as when and what to ask.

> I learned that every word I choose, every motion I make with my hands, body and eyes impact a therapeutic relationship.

> I have become so much more aware of my interaction style as an interviewer. . . . Awareness of topics such as self-disclosure and termination helped me realize how I need to deal with these issues in order to create and maintain a positive therapeutic relationship.

Students are extremely positive about having the opportunity to meet and interview guest speakers living with disabilities:

> The guest speakers offered a wonderful opportunity to reflect [on] and examine my own perception of disability as well as their own. The interview questions were a great idea to teach us how to think about the individual, think on our feet, be reflective and intuitive.

> I enjoyed the problem list aspect of the interview and speaker assignment. It is a useful tool to understand or examine the perspective of a person with a particular illness or disability in the areas of occupational performance. It encourages one to consider all aspects of one's life, rather than focusing on a single performance area.

> Interviewing guest speakers gave me a wealth of knowledge. Hearing good questions other students came up with was very useful.

On cultural sensitivity, students wrote:

> I feel that building a respect for the power of reflection was important for me. The course offered great discussions on cultural sensitivity.

> I'm pleased to say the course made me more aware of people's differences in beliefs and attitudes–and to respect that. I'd like to think I'm more culturally sensitive now.

Students' ratings of the course on the American Occupational Therapy Association Fieldwork Evaluation Forms, completed following their fieldwork placements, ranged from 3 to 5 (on a scale of 0 to 5) regarding how well the course prepared them for their fieldwork. Although we did not perform a formal analysis of the ratings, it was noted that students in psychosocial settings gave higher ratings for the course than those in settings for people with physical disabilities, and those who had the opportunity to interview clients reported that the course prepared them very well.

Another perspective on the value of the course comes from the guest speakers themselves. Two guest speakers who have participated in the course for several years were asked what was in it for them, what it was like for them to come back year after year and talk to our students. S. said:

> I enjoy it. I believe in what you're doing. I've seen what a difference a good OT can make. I told your students about my buddy, an OT, who figured out a better shower seat for me when mine wasn't working.

S. takes a proprietary approach to students:

> I like to encourage them. They're the next inventors and discoverers.

When asked about his experience speaking with students, S. responded:

> Oh, I enjoy it; I get a kick out of it. They're always interested; they listen hard. It's always interesting talking to intelligent people.

S. is a university graduate interested in reading philosophy, as well as a soccer coach who loves to travel to Italy with his team. He has been through some very difficult times as a result of his spinal cord injury and recent hospitalizations with ulcers, which may have prompted him to add:

> These men and women [the students] are our hope for a lot of people. I tell them not to be afraid of situations that look as if they're hopeless, because nothing is hopeless and there are always ways to make things better.

When B. was asked what it was like to come back year after year to talk to our students, he said:

> I like to talk to them and answer their questions. I want students to know there is life after a spinal cord injury. You can do things and have fun. I want them to see that life has gone on for me and for others.

Several months after the course was over, one author happened to overhear two students having a conversation about cultural sensitivity. One student said: "I learned most about other people's perspectives when we met those guest speakers with AIDS in [the Interactive Clinical Reasoning course]." The other student replied:

> Yeah, that was the first time I had knowingly met anyone with AIDS. I'm sure I had met someone before, but I didn't know it. It made him a real person and there he was sitting there and it wasn't just a textbook diagno-

sis. Of course, I knew they were real people, but this really brought it home to me–face to face talking to him.

The guiding philosophy and tenets of a course to teach interactive clinical reasoning have been presented. Content and assignments have been described in the hope that educators may find this a useful approach for the development of students' skills, techniques, and sensitivity when interacting with people with disabilities. Rigorous reflection on their own perspectives, coupled with a thorough examination of the interview process with people who live with disability, provides students with a foundation for understanding others. We hope this foundation will establish in students a desire to be introspective in their future practice and to continue to deliberate on their interactions with clients.

REFERENCES

American Occupational Therapy Association. (1996). Position paper: Providing services for persons with HIV/AIDS and their caregivers. *The reference manual of the official documents of the American Occupational Therapy Association* (7th ed.), (pp. 237-241).

Bailey, D. M. (2000). Introducing an awareness of cultural diversity into an established curriculum. In P. Crist (ed.), *Innovations in occupational therapy education 2000* (pp. 134-145). Bethesda, MD: AOTA.

Barris, R., Oakley, F., & Kielhofner, G. (1988). The Role Checklist. In B. Hemphill (ed.), *Mental health assessment in occupational therapy: An integrated approach to the evaluative process* (pp. 73-91). Thorofare, NJ: Slack Inc.

Charmaz, K. (1991). Translating graduate qualitative methods into undergraduate teaching: Intensive interviewing as a case example. *Teaching Sociology, 19*, 384-395.

Cohn, E. S. (1989). Fieldwork education: Shaping a foundation for clinical reasoning. *American Journal of Occupational Therapy, 43*, 240-244.

Cohn, E. S. (1991). Clinical reasoning: Explicating complexity. *American Journal of Occupational Therapy, 45*, 969-971.

Cohn, E. S. (1993, December). Inquiring minds: A curriculum designed to facilitate clinical reasoning. *Education Special Interest Section Newsletter, 3*, 1-4.

Coles, R. (1989). *The call of stories*. Cambridge, MA: Harvard University Press.

Crepeau, E. B. (1991). Achieving intersubjective understanding: Examples from an occupational therapy treatment session. *American Journal of Occupational Therapy, 45*, 1016-1025.

Davis, C. M. (1998). *Patient practitioner interaction: An experiential manual for developing the art of health care* (3rd ed.). Thorofare, NJ: Slack Inc.

Emener, W. G. (1991). Empowerment in rehabilitation: An empowerment philosophy for rehabilitation in the 20th century. *Journal of Rehabilitation, 57*, 229-34.

Fleming, M. H. (1991). The therapist with a three-track mind. *American Journal of Occupational Therapy, 45*, 1007-1014.

Gardner, H. (1985). *Frames of mind: The theory of multiple intelligences.* New York: Basic Books.

Howe, M., & Schwartzberg, S. (1995). *A functional approach to group work in occupational therapy* (2nd ed.). Philadelphia: Lippincott.

Jackson, J. (1995). Sexual orientation: Its relevance to occupational science and the practice of occupational therapy. *American Journal of Occupational Therapy, 49,* 669-679.

Kautzmann, L. N. (1993). Linking patient and family stories to caregivers' use of clinical reasoning. *American Journal of Occupational Therapy, 47,* 169-173.

Kielhofner, G., Henry, A., & Walens, D. (1989). *A user's guide to the Occupational Performance History.* Rockville, MD: AOTA.

Maholick, L., & Turner, D. (1979). Termination: That difficult farewell. *American Journal of Psychotherapy, 33,* 103-109.

Martin, K., & Berchule, C. (1988). The effect of dying and death on therapists. In *Community programs for the health impaired elderly.* Binghamton, NY: The Haworth Press, Inc.

Mattingly, C. (1991). The narrative nature of clinical reasoning. *American Journal of Occupational Therapy, 45,* 998-1005.

Mattingly, C. (1992). Clinical reasoning. Unpublished manuscript.

Mattingly, C., & Fleming, M. H. (1994). *Clinical reasoning: Forms of inquiry in a therapeutic practice.* Philadelphia: F. A. Davis.

McIntosh, P. (1989, July/August). White privilege: Unpacking the invisible knapsack. *Peace and Freedom,* 10-12.

Mishler, E. (1986). *Research interviewing: Context and narrative.* Cambridge, MA: Harvard University Press.

Murphy, B. C., & Dillon, C. (1998). *Interviewing in action: Process and practice.* Pacific Grove, CA: Brooks/Cole Publishing Co. (Videotape and text).

Neistadt, M. E. (1987). The classroom as clinic: A model for teaching clinical reasoning in occupational therapy education. *American Journal of Occupational Therapy, 41,* 631-637.

Neistadt, M. E. (1992). The classroom as clinic: Applications for a method of teaching clinical reasoning. *American Journal of Occupational Therapy, 46,* 814-819.

Neistadt, M. E. (1996). Teaching strategies for the development of clinical reasoning. *American Journal of Occupational Therapy, 50,* 676-684.

Neistadt, M. E. (1998). Teaching clinical reasoning as a thinking frame. *American Journal of Occupational Therapy, 52,* 221-229.

Neistadt, M. E., Wight, J., & Mulligan, S. E. (1998). Clinical reasoning case studies as teaching tools. *American Journal of Occupational Therapy, 52,* 125-132.

Parham, D. (1987). Nationally speaking–toward professionalism: The reflective therapist. *American Journal of Occupational Therapy, 41,* 555-561.

Peloquin, S. M. (1989). Sustaining the art of practice in occupational therapy. *American Journal of Occupational Therapy, 43,* 219-226.

Peloquin, S. M. (1995). The fullness of empathy: Reflections and illustrations. *American Journal of Occupational Therapy, 49,* 24-31.

Peloquin, S. M., & Babola, K. A. (1996). Making of a clinical climate in the classroom. *American Journal of Occupational Therapy, 50,* 894-898.

Rogers, J. C. (1983). Eleanor Clarke Slagle lectureship 1983–Clinical reasoning: The ethics, science, and art. *American Journal of Occupational Therapy, 37,* 601-616.

Schell, B. A. (1998). Clinical reasoning: The basis of practice. In M. E. Neistadt & E. B. Crepeau (eds.), *Willard and Spackman's occupational therapy* (9th ed.). Philadelphia: Lippincott.

Schell, B. A., & Cervero, R. M. (1993). Clinical reasoning in occupational therapy: An integrative review. *American Journal of Occupational Therapy, 47,* 605-610.

Schwartz, K. B. (1991). Clinical reasoning and new ideas on intelligence: Implications for teaching and learning. *American Journal of Occupational Therapy, 45,* 1033-1037.

Spencer, J., Krefting, L., & Mattingly, C. (1993). Incorporation of ethnographic methods in occupational therapy assessment. *American Journal of Occupational Therapy, 47,* 303-309.

Tickle-Degnen, L. (1995). Therapeutic rapport. In C. A. Trombly (ed.), *Occupational therapy for physical dysfunction* (pp. 277-286). Baltimore, MD: Williams & Wilkins.

VanLeit, B. (1995). Using the case study method to develop clinical reasoning skills in problem-based learning. *American Journal of Occupational Therapy, 49,* 9-353.

Zola, I. K. (1993). Self, identity and the naming question: Reflections on the language of disability. *Social Science and Medicine, 36,* 167-173.

APPENDIX A

Interactive Clinical Reasoning Course Objectives

By the end of the course, students will be able to:

(a) Simultaneously observe and interact with others, as evidenced by written analysis of peer interview (which has been videotaped) and performance during guest interviews.

(b) Identify and interpret personal responses to others' behaviors, as evidenced by written analysis of peer and culture interviews and oral reporting in small groups following guest interviews.

(c) Modify interactive style in response to others, as evidenced by written analysis of videotaped peer interviews, performance during guest interviews, and performance during small group exercises.

(d) Analyze interactive style in relation to therapeutic use of self, as evidenced by written analysis of performance during guest interviews, performance in small group exercises, and analysis of self assignment.

(e) Understand how values affect therapeutic relationships, as evidenced by written analysis of guest interviews, interview with person from a different culture, written analysis and discussion of readings, and analysis of self assignment.

(f) Identify potential domains of concern for occupational therapy based on consumers' perspectives, as evidenced by written analysis and discussion of guest interviews and readings.

(g) Understand human behavior in the context of sociocultural systems, as evidenced by written analysis and discussion of all interviews, assignments, and readings.

APPENDIX B

Analysis of Self

ASSIGNMENT: Analysis of personal identities and implications for learning and practice.

GOALS: We ask you to reflect on your own social identities and the meanings you and society attach to them. The goal of the assignment is to help you understand how these factors influence your ability to engage in culturally relevant and meaningful occupations, and your therapeutic use of self.

DIRECTIONS: In each social identity category listed below, describe your position and reflect on its implications. For example, if you are privileged in one of the categories, what, most likely, have you taken for granted? Where you may be subordinate or disadvantaged, how do you cope and what have you learned about yourself and your response to oppression? In each case, what are the challenges you are likely to encounter when developing your awareness, knowledge, and skills to become an occupational therapist? What do you need to learn?

NOTE: This form is for your personal use only, and you will not be asked to show it to peers or instructors. You have control over what and how much information you choose to disclose and with whom you wish to share. Please save this form for use in other courses.

Age:
Race:
Nationality/Ethnicity:
Language facility:
Socioeconomic class:
Sex:
Religion:
Sexual orientation:
Disabilities:
Health:
Physical size and appearance:
Education level:
Occupation/occupational roles:
Mannerisms and styles of presenting and interacting with others:

[Adapted from: Jean Wu (1998). *Your diversity/cultural competence challenge.* Tufts University-Boston School of Occupational Therapy Workshop on Engaging Diversity in Preparation for Practice.]

APPENDIX C

Cultural Awareness Assignment

The aim is for students to think about the progression that can be made from being afraid or ignorant of others' cultural differences -> to making an effort to learn about differences -> to a sincere curiosity and wanting to know about another's culture -> to ultimately celebrating and enjoying another's diversity. Finally, we want students to think about the relationship of diversity to occupational functioning and the therapeutic relationship.

Exercise

*In pairs, interview a classmate to *really* discover how they construct the meaning of the sick role. Questions may center around:
> how illness is handled in their family
> what is defined as a severe illness
> how do people in their family behave in relation to illness (both the person who is sick and the caretakers)?

*Think about what your interviewee might want from a caregiver. Try these ideas out with the interviewee and get feedback on your perceptions.

*Allow 15 minutes for the first interview.

*Switch roles and partners, so that everyone gets a chance to take both roles.

*Repeat the interview for 15 minutes.

*In the whole group, share findings about what people want from caregivers and what that means for students in their future role as therapists. (Would they be able to provide that? Take that role? Be comfortable with that behavior?)

The goal is to help students be more astute at figuring out the ways clients want practitioners to interact with them.

Parameters for Adapting
Journal Writing Activities

Rick Hobbs, MA, OTR/L
Aimee J. Luebben, EdD, OTR/L, FAOTA

SUMMARY. The purpose of this article is to discuss journal writing parameters, which have proven useful in shaping student journal assignments. In a qualitative audit of journal writing activities currently utilized in an occupational therapy curriculum at a midwestern university, the authors used four parameters–focus, temporality, feedback, and sharing–to analyze five student journal strategies: Video Journal, OT/OTA Collaborative Fieldwork Journal, Course Objectives Journal, Subject-Specific Journal, and Activity Response Journal. A student exemplar follows the parameter analysis for each journal writing strategy. Various outcome evaluation methods show journal writing activities to be valuable tools in a curriculum that emphasizes reflection, critical thinking skills, and learner-centered educational approaches. Adaptable by means of the four parameters, these five generic student journal activities can be easily implemented in a variety of courses, allowing for development of professional attitudes, relationships, and skills. *[Article copies available for a fee from The Haworth Document Delivery Service: 1-800-HAWORTH. E-mail address: <getinfo@haworthpressinc.com> Website: <http://www.HaworthPress.com>* © 2001 by The Haworth Press, Inc. All rights reserved.]

Rick Hobbs is Assistant Professor and Advising Coordinator, Occupational Therapy Program, University of Southern Indiana, Evansville, IN 44714.

Aimee J. Luebben is Associate Professor and Director, Occupational Therapy Program, University of Southern Indiana, Evansville, IN.

[Haworth co-indexing entry note]: "Parameters for Adapting Journal Writing Activities." Hobbs, Rick, and Aimee J. Luebben. Co-published simultaneously in *Occupational Therapy in Health Care* (The Haworth Press, Inc.) Vol. 15, No. 1/2, 2001, pp. 47-55; and: *Education for Occupational Therapy in Health Care: Strategies for the New Millennium* (eds: Patricia Crist, and Marjorie Scaffa) The Haworth Press, Inc., 2001, pp. 47-55. Single or multiple copies of this article are available for a fee from The Haworth Document Delivery Service [1-800-HAWORTH, 9:00 a.m. - 5:00 p.m. (EST). E-mail address: getinfo@haworthpressinc.com].

KEYWORDS. Education, student journals, journal writing

For purposes of education, defining a journal writing activity may seem a perplexing task. Although many have contributed ideas (Black, Sileo, & Prater, 2000; Hodges, 1996; Patton et al., 1997; Tryssenaar, 1995), two characteristics do seem to hold fast: journal writing is done at a relatively set frequency and includes a relatively robust subjective component involving an individual's ideas, thoughts, and reflections. The authors of this article do not wish to argue the efficacy of journal writing as an educational activity since numerous papers have documented journal writing efficacy in terms of facilitating reflection and critical thinking (Black et al., 2000), knowledge construction (Hughes, Kooy, & Kanevsky, 1997), communication between student and instructor (Goldsby & Cozza, 1998), and writing skills (Manning, 1999). Rather, the purpose of this article is to discuss parameters of journal writing, exploring how student journal activities may be adapted to fit various pedagogical uses. Patton et al. (1997) have noted a lack of empirical data supporting the efficacy of journal writing in the educational process; however, such studies may be difficult to undertake until the full breadth and intricacy of the journaling tool are more fully explored. Journal writing activities can be potentially effective, but not until this educational strategy is more fully understood in terms of its various parameters and situational uses.

METHODS

Focus, temporality, feedback, and sharing are four parameters that can help educators conceptualize and adapt a journal writing assignment to a specific pedagogical purpose. The focus of any journal writing activity involves two aspects: entry type and domain. Entry type refers to journal format, which is commonly categorized into single-, double-, and triple-entry. The single-entry journal (i.e., one person writing one entry) is a common type of journal writing; however, dividing the format to link journal entries in combinations (e.g., double- and triple-entry journals) works effectively. Double- and triple-entry journals can be written by an individual or more than one student. Domain refers to the classic hierarchical categorization of educational objectives, developed originally by Bloom, Englehart, Furst, Hill, and Krathwohl (1956), into three domains: cognitive, affective, and psychomotor. Student occupations, those everyday activities in which the individual in an occupational therapy student role participates, can be classified into these domains. Appropriate journal writing student occupations include knowing, comprehending, applying, analyzing, synthesizing, and evaluating in the cognitive domain and receiving, responding, and valuing in the affective domain.

The temporality parameter entails a blending of the frequency of the entries, duration of the journal writing activity, and interval between entries. The frequency of the entries can range from daily, several times per week, weekly, linked with the occurrence of specific events to "as needed," whereas duration of the journal writing activity can vary from year-long, semester-long, fieldwork-long, the time span of a group or project as needed. The time interval between entries can range from allowing the student to set the interval to prescribing a set length of time between entries. While the time interval between entries may not seem of particular importance, assigning a three-day interval between journal entries may facilitate additional reflection on an assigned course topic.

The feedback parameter indicates the degree to which another person (usually the instructor) responds to the student's entries and the timeliness of the response. During the design of a student journal assignment, an instructor might work through some of the following questions: Are queries to the instructor encouraged or discouraged? Would the instructor like the student to engage in a dialog by responding to the faculty member's comments? Could an entry lead to face-to-face discussion, or even class discussion? Is venting or speculating allowed, without expectation (or fear) of the instructor commenting (unless asked)? The question of the degree of feedback also entails the timeliness of the feedback. Will the student submit the journal weekly, every other week, with each individual entry, at the conclusion of a project, or at the end of the semester? Given the assigned focus of the journal activity, how timely does the instructor's response need to be?

To what degree journal entries are shared is another important parameter. The entries can be shared with other students to facilitate further exploration or to communicate provocative ideas, either in class discussion or on an individual basis. The information within a journal may be shared with other faculty members or shared only within a given group of students. The journal writing activity may also be assigned with the stipulation that the individual student's entries will be read only by the instructor responsible for the course. Any information imparted would then be kept in confidence–possibly encouraging the student to address thoughts and feelings he or she may otherwise feel less comfortable sharing. Prudence and principle dictate that the degree to which the journal entries are to be shared should be made clear when the journal writing activity is assigned–and adhered to rigidly.

RESULTS

In a qualitative audit of journal writing activities currently utilized in five courses within the occupational therapy curriculum, the authors used the four parameters—focus, temporality, feedback, and sharing—to analyze five student journal strategies: Video Journal, OT/OTA Collaborative Fieldwork Journal, Course Objectives Journal, Subject-Specific Journal, and Activity Response Journal. A student exemplar follows the analysis of individual journal writing strategies.

The focus of the Video Journal is integration of new knowledge gained from assigned videotapes viewed outside class, information from reading assignments and class discussions, and reflection on ideas, concerns, and beliefs. Student occupations emphasized in this single-entry journaling assignment include comprehending and applying in the cognitive domain and responding and valuing in the affective domain. Temporality is addressed by having students complete one journal entry after viewing each video assigned. Frequency of entries equals the number of assigned videos; however, duration and interval are not specified. Feedback occurs when the instructor collects student video journals at the end of the school term, comments on student insights, and answers queries. Writing the following example, a student shares with the instructor this information:

> Watching this video, I realized that I have already learned so much about occupational therapy. At the same time, I know that I still have a lot to learn. Of course the learning process should never really end, should it?

The focus of the OT/OTA Collaborative Fieldwork Journal is cooperation between paired occupational therapy practitioner students during a Level I fieldwork practicum. During the long drive to and from an early intervention fieldwork site, two students, an occupational therapy major and an occupational therapy assistant major, complete double-entry journals by responding in the left column to identical writing prompts (written by the fieldwork educator prior to the scheduled day). The pair exchange journals and, in the right column, write comments on each other's responses. This fieldwork journal emphasizes three student occupations (applying, analyzing, and synthesizing) in the cognitive domain and two student occupations (valuing and organizing values) in the affective domain. For this student journal assignment, temporality is specified: frequency is twice per assigned fieldwork day with students completing one set of prompts before the fieldwork experience begins and the second set after the final visit of the day, duration is two songs playing sequentially on the car radio, and interval equals the length of time between scheduled fieldwork days. To address feedback, the fieldwork educator collects student journals after each scheduled fieldwork day to review student responses and write prompts for the next session. In this case, student journals are not graded. Fieldwork practicum students share their thoughts with each other during the day scheduled for fieldwork and with the fieldwork educator at the end of each session. The occupational therapy student was the primary respondent in Table 1 with the occupational therapy assistant student in the collaborator role.

For the Course Objectives Journal, students focus on a concept, fact, or idea addressed in the week's learning objectives in the first column, and in the second column address their thoughts, reflections, and speculations on the significance of the concept, fact, or idea described. Each column of this double-entry journal provides an emphasis on a different domain: the first column emphasizes the cognitive domain, primarily the two student occupations of knowing and comprehending, and the second column emphasizes three student occupations (receiving, responding, and valuing) in the affective domain. The temporality of this assignment requires students to complete two double-entries for each of the first nine class sessions with one-half of the double-entry to be made immediately following the class session. To promote reflection, the second half of the double-entry must be completed no sooner than three days following the class session. Feedback for this assignment includes collecting and reading journals randomly, and assigning points. Students share their journals with the instructor, the instructor's representative, or fellow students. Table 2 provides an example of a student describing a set of neuroscience course objectives in the first column with two dated entries reflecting on new knowledge in the second column.

The focus of the Subject-Specific Journal is reflection on a realization, observation, interaction, situation, relationship, incident, or dilemma–social, psychological, ethical, sensorimotor, environmental, and/or educational in nature. The instructor invites students to feel free to vent occasionally, advises that they may not come to a conclusion with their thoughts, and invites questions. Although students utilize three student occupations (analyzing, synthesizing, and evaluating) in the cognitive domain, the primary emphasis of this student journal is the affective domain (valuing, organizing values, and internalizing values). Temporality for this assignment includes (a) frequency: three times per week for the semester and (b) duration: the instructor indicates a preference for entries no longer than one page, but permits longer entries if thoughts occasionally move students to greater lengths. The interval between entries is left to each student's discretion. Students submit journals with pre-specified numbers of entries on seven occasions during the semester, and the instructor assigns points for student engagement and clarity. In the following exemplar, a student shared with the instructor:

TABLE 1. OT/OTA Collaborative Fieldwork Journal: Day 2 P.M.

Writing Prompt: What interested you most about today and how are you going to further your own development in that area?

OT Student	OTA Student
The vision problems with the first child were interesting. I wonder what exactly his world looks like. To develop this I could read upon vision cuts and how they could present themselves or about how both eyes may not be in line.	He was very interesting. I think it would be neat to see his world too.

The other night I watched a special on TV about how car manufacturers design seats. It was interesting to see that our population is getting larger and larger (and I don't mean taller). The program showed how they scan in a person's picture into a computer and the computer calculated the length of different body parts in different positions. I was fascinated by how much thought goes into making a car's interior ergonomic. I have a strong interest in ergonomics. Can you work for a company doing work station alterations and treat the employees with injuries from the job without having an ergonomics certification and without upsetting the workers' comp programs?

For the Activity Response Journal, the focus is student engagement in sessions of sensorimotor awareness, psychosocial awareness, or environmental awareness and then reflection on the subjective experience as well as observations related to the course concepts. This single-entry assignment emphasizes three student occupations (comprehending, applying, and analyzing) in the cognitive domain and receiving and responding, two student occupations in the affective domain. Although the instructor assigns a specific journal writing assignment on the day of the activity, the only temporality aspect is the instructor's preset collection dates for student journals. Sharing takes place between the student and instructor; faculty feedback includes clarity of thought and assignment engagement. Reflecting on a trip to a union local for a course on work and productive activities, a student wrote:

A few key points Mr. C. illustrated made me realize my one experience with the union should not be utilized to draw a conclusion about the un-

TABLE 2. Neuroscience Journal

List the various functions the brain is expected to perform:	
• Perceive and associate stimulation • Regulate body function • Maintain (survival drive) • Learn • React	Sept. 1: This knowledge makes me aware of how important the brain is to every action of every individual. It also enlightens me for when I will begin dealing with neurology patients. Realizing the types of functions affected by a brain injury, can give me as an OTS great insight for intervention. Sept. 5: This makes me wonder why people damage their brain by consuming large amounts of alcohol and using different drugs, when most are mature enough and intelligent to know what can happen to themselves when they destroy their brain by these actions.

ion in general. One of these key points was that often the stereotypes that accompany the union are directly related to poor leadership. In my experience, there was no distinct leader saying okay, enough is enough. Another point Mr. C. made was that it would be in the union members' best interest if all members satisfactorily performed their jobs to ensure optimum productivity, so why wouldn't they? Good point, in reflection, I find that many times when people degrade union workers, it is due to a negative experience like mine, which does not accurately describe all union workers. The union could utilize an occupational therapist in many ways. The therapist would have to possess the ability to communicate with a manual labor worker and be extremely flexible. Obvious ways would include ergonomics in the workplace, work hardening, and wellness.

DISCUSSION

Essentially, focus, temporality, feedback, and sharing are four parameters that can determine the degree to which a given journal writing activity addresses the instructor's intent. Additionally, these parameters may be adjusted within a specific assigned activity. A journal writing assignment, designed to facilitate a student's awareness of environmental issues, may be reduced in required frequency of entries once the desired behavior has been established and sufficiently reinforced. A student journal designed to provide topics for class discussion may be stopped once students feel comfortable in spontaneously offering topics. Again, the parameters provide a means of adapting the journaling activity towards a given goal, and may be adjusted as goals are achieved.

Overall, students have been receptive to journaling even though difficulties have arisen in implementing various journal writing activities. Although many have commented that they initially perceived the activity as "busy work," as the activity proceeded–and the goals of the activity became more realistically apparent to participants–they acknowledged the value in the activity as an educational tool. For other students, a particular activity was the first time they had experienced journaling with pointed feedback, with the assurance of confidentiality, and/or within the particular format assigned. Building trust of participating students when confidentiality is required in the particular journal writing activity's focus takes time, diligence, and patience–and has to be earned. Lapses, or even rumors of lapses, can be devastating, as current students often rely on the previous year's participants for assurances and mentoring. Assisting the individual student in honing his or her focus can also be an issue. The student may not realize how an assigned journal writing activity has been fine-tuned to fit the pedagogical needs of a course. Often, patience and more frequent feedback are required at the beginning of a journaling activity. Grading criteria for journal writing can vary greatly across activities and very much depend upon the focus of a given activity.

The Video Journal, Course Objectives Journal, Subject-Specific Journal, and Activity Response Journal have undergone summative student and faculty evaluation via the quality improvement process. Students indicated in the spring 2000 *Quality Improvement Survey* that journaling was an effective learning strategy in becoming a reflective practitioner. In the fall 2000 Quality Improvement Meeting, reflection (accomplished through journaling) followed evaluation skills and "thinking on feet" as the third curriculum strength students listed. Practicum students wrote in the *Evaluation of the Level I Fieldwork Site* that the OT/OTA Collaborative Fieldwork Journal offered a low-key get-acquainted strategy, provided a less scary communication pattern, developed an early support system, offered organizational strategies, helped design future learning strategies, provided insight into the affective aspect of learning, and promoted team building.

For the instructor seeking alternatives to traditional teaching methods, journal writing is a valuable tool. Adaptable in focus, temporality, feedback, and sharing, student journals can allow for the development of professional attitudes, relationships, and skills. Journal writing activities have permitted the practice and development of related skills, such as exploration and concise expression of concepts, feelings, concerns, ideas, and descriptions. In addition, journal writing strategies have helped establish a running dialogue between the individual student and the instructor, assisting the educator in becoming acquainted with the student's needs, hopes, fears, and circumstances, and potentially helping to establish a mentoring relationship.

REFERENCES

Black, R. S., Sileo, T. W., & Prater, M. A. (2000). Learning journals, self-reflection, and university students' changing perceptions. *Action in Teacher Education, 21*, 71-89.

Bloom, B. S., Englehart, M., Furst, E., Hill, W., & Krathwohl, D. (Eds.). (1956). *Taxonomy of educational objectives–Volume 1: The cognitive domain.* New York: McKay.

Goldsby, D. S., & Cozza, B. (1998). Using reflective journals in college education courses. *Kappa Delta Pi Record, 34*, 112-113.

Hodges, H. F. (1996). Journal writing as a mode of thinking for RN-BSN students: A leveled approach to learning to listen to self and others. *Journal of Nursing Education, 35*, 137-141.

Hughes, H. W., Kooy, M., & Kanevsky, L. (1997). Dialogic reflection and journaling. *The Clearing House, 70*, 187-190.

Manning, M. (1999). Too many journals? *Teaching PreK-8, 30*, 89-90.

Patton, J. G., Woods, S. J., Agarenzo, T., Brubaker, C., Metcalf, T., & Sherrer, L. (1997). Enhancing the clinical practicum experience through journal writing. *Journal of Nursing Education, 36*, 238-240.

Tryssenaar, J. (1995). Interactive journals: An educational strategy to promote reflection. *American Journal of Occupational Therapy, 49*, 695-702.

FIELDWORK EDUCATION

The Reindeer of Hope:
An Occupational Therapy Program in a Homeless Shelter

Anne Shordike, MOT, OTR/L
Donna Howell, OTS

SUMMARY. This article describes a successfully designed and implemented program created for mentally ill homeless men by Level II occupational therapy students from Eastern Kentucky University. Outcomes for the clients, the staff and the students were extremely positive and have contributed to the appreciation and acceptance of occupational therapy as a discipline that can contribute to the health of this underserved population. This model demonstrates the effectiveness of University sponsored fieldwork in introducing occupational therapy to the community, creating awareness of what occupational therapy has to offer and developing a climate to bring

---

Anne Shordike is Assistant Professor, Department of Occupational Therapy, Eastern Kentucky University, Richmond, KY.

Donna Howell is also affiliated with Eastern Kentucky University, Richmond, KY 40475.

[Haworth co-indexing entry note]: "The Reindeer of Hope: An Occupational Therapy Program in a Homeless Shelter." Shordike, Anne, and Donna Howell. Co-published simultaneously in *Occupational Therapy in Health Care* (The Haworth Press, Inc.) Vol. 15, No. 1/2, 2001, pp. 57-68; and: *Education for Occupational Therapy in Health Care: Strategies for the New Millennium* (eds: Patricia Crist, and Marjorie Scaffa) The Haworth Press, Inc., 2001, pp. 57-68. Single or multiple copies of this article are available for a fee from The Haworth Document Delivery Service [1-800-HAWORTH, 9:00 a.m. - 5:00 p.m. (EST). E-mail address: getinfo@haworthpressinc.com].

57

needed services to clients and provide community-based employment for occupational therapists. *[Article copies available for a fee from The Haworth Document Delivery Service: 1-800-HAWORTH. E-mail address: <getinfo@ haworthpressinc.com> Website: <http://www.HaworthPress.com> © 2001 by The Haworth Press, Inc. All rights reserved.]*

KEYWORDS. Education, community, mental health

INTRODUCTION

The Occupational Therapy Department at Eastern Kentucky University has utilized nontraditional, community-based, Level I fieldwork education for the past decade. Several of these community service-based placements have been described by Rydeen, Kautzmann, Cowan, and Benzing (1995). The development of Level I placements at the Hope Center, a homeless shelter for men in Lexington, Kentucky, is detailed in Scaffa, Brownson, and Shordike (2001). The success of these faculty-facilitated experiences at the homeless shelter lay the groundwork for the introduction of Level II occupational therapy students at this facility.

In the Fall of 1999 Eastern Kentucky University began a level II fieldwork program at the Hope Center. Two students who were supervised by faculty created an occupational therapy program within the existing mental health programs at the center. One purpose of this particular Level II program was to give the students an opportunity to create a program from the ground up, from documentation through program development and implementation, to prepare students for "the new demands of community health roles" (Scaffa, Brownson, & Shordike, 2001). Another purpose was to explore the effectiveness of introducing occupational therapy to this facility through University/community agency collaboration. The purpose of the living skills program for the participants was to increase their independence, productivity, and satisfaction in valued life roles.

REVIEW OF THE LITERATURE

The increase in the homeless population is well documented although statistics regarding the actual number of homeless people differ, depending on the time or manner in which they are counted. The Interagency Council on the Homeless (1994) found that twelve million adults in the United States have been homeless at some time in their lives. Several studies have found a relationship between substance abuse, mental illness, and homelessness. Approximately fifty-six percent of the homeless have substance abuse problems, and twelve to twenty-five percent of these individuals are considered to be dually diagnosed (Cnaan & Blankertz, 1993). One-third to one-half of the single, adult homeless suffer from a severe or persistent mental illness (Kavanagh & Fares, 1995; Kiesler, 1991; Kondratas, 1991; Lehman & Cordray, 1995). Mental illness and its symptoms, such as hallucinations, anxiety, depression, antisocial or aggressive behaviors, may prevent people from carrying out essential daily life tasks (Fischer & Breakey, 1991; National Coalition for the Homeless, 1999). Studies also suggest that individuals with severe mental illness are at higher risk for becoming homeless and remaining homeless longer, due to their deficits in independent living skills (Dennis, Levine, & Osher, 1991; Fischer & Breakey, 1991; National Coalition for the Homeless, 1999). Lloyd and Samra (1996) state that the emphasis of treatment for the homeless mentally ill should be on promoting wellness by optimizing independent functioning through skills training. They go on to state that the intervention should focus on the desired functional outcome rather than diagnosis or symptoms.

Occupational therapy involvement with the homeless has begun to emerge in practice and the literature during the past decade. Drake (1992) describes occupational therapy services implemented through a fieldwork program in a center for homeless children. Barth (1995) discusses occupational therapy intervention in a community agency for the homeless. She considers roles occupational therapy can take beyond direct treatment. Marks (1997) suggests a consultation role for occupational therapists working with homeless agencies. Kavanagh and Fares (1995) use the Model of Human Occupation as a way to design interventions for homeless individuals. Heubner and Tryssenaar (1996) describe a Level I fieldwork placement that supports the transition of occupational therapy to community-based mental health service delivery. Kannenberg and Boyer (1997) implemented an occupational therapy program for homeless youths to address their developmental and functional deficits. These models and studies demonstrate the involvement of occupational therapists with the homeless and speak to occupational therapy's social vision (Townsend, 1993) and commitment to community living and social justice (Mitchell & Jones, 1997).

PROGRAM DEVELOPMENT

The Hope Center is a 116-bed non-profit facility that provides services to all of Lexington's homeless population; however, the focus of the residential component is to serve single, adult males. Men may stay overnight or they may become involved in the day programs offered at the Center. These programs include a Mental Health Program, a Substance Abuse Recovery Program, and a Hispanic Program. A Mobile Outreach Program and a Housing Support Program serve clients in the community. Level I Occupational Therapy students have been involved in all of these programs since 1997 (Scaffa, Brownson, & Shordike, 2001).

The Level II occupational therapy students created a program for the residential mental health clients, including treatment groups, individual interventions, and documentation. Assignments included development of a screening tool and treatment plan format. They were also required to produce a final project that would benefit the clients, the agency, and their own professional development. They were expected to participate in measurement of outcomes for the program. They received assistance from Level I students one day a week and participated in the supervision of the Level I students. The fifteen participants in the program were all men, aged 20 to 65. Each of them had an Axis I diagnosis, including Major Depression, Bipolar Affective Disorder, and several of the Schizophrenias. Two carried a diagnosis of Borderline Personality Disorder, five had concomitant medical problems, and seven had identified substance abuse issues.

The students created a screening tool, based on performance areas, to identify individual participant priorities, skills, and strengths. From the screen, they proceeded to a more specifically targeted evaluation and treatment planning process. Some of the assessments used were the Kohlman Evaluation of Living Skills (Kohlman-Thompson, 1992), the Allen Cognitive Level Test (Allen, 1985), the Role Checklist (Barris, Oakley, & Kielhofner, 1988), the Bay Area Functional Performance Evaluation (Williams, & Bloomer, 1987), and the Canadian Occupational Performance Measure (Law, Baptiste, Carswell-Opzoomer, McColl, Polatajko, & Pollack, 1994). These evaluations identified individual needs in the areas of self-care, instrumental activities of daily living, productive and leisure occupations, perceived self-efficacy, and interpersonal skills. The treatment plan was based on the evaluations and functional observation; when completed it was discussed with, agreed to, and signed by the client. Ten of the fifteen individuals who participated in the needs assessment and treatment planning process became consistent program participants; the others were discharged by the center or by their own choosing.

PROGRAM DESCRIPTION

A program was created that addressed the individual needs of the clients within groups that taught skills necessary for independence in their valued life roles. Thematic topics such as personal hygiene, clothing care, money management, leisure, and work were graded from basic to complex as the weeks progressed. For example, during the clothing care unit, participants learned how to use the washing machine and dryer to clean their clothes and also how to sew on buttons and mend their clothes. During the work unit, the clients learned about interview appropriate dress and behavior, practiced interviews and gave each other feedback, and filled out time cards and job applications. Each week the clients planned a meal, shopped for groceries, and prepared the meal. For Thanksgiving, they invited staff and friends to join them. All of the food related activities included nutrition education, money management, and social skills.

THE REINDEER OF HOPE

The students responded to the clients' success in and commitment to the program by collaborating with them to design a holiday workshop that produced and sold log reindeer. The participants had previously demonstrated an interest in and capacity for woodworking while participating in a birdhouse building project. In order to implement the reindeer workshop the students had to negotiate workshop space within the center and write a proposal for approval by staff and the Board of Directors of the Hope Center.

Once the reindeer were designed, with the help of a client, job notices were posted in the meeting areas for the mental health clients. Each prospective employee filled out a job application and went through an interview process. The job descriptions were specific to each individual's desires, skill level, and cognitive level. Training in safe tool use was required and provided. Some of the men were involved in power tool use; not all of the men used all of the tools. Others worked in assembly with hand tools. Other types of jobs included finishing, quality control, setting up, and cleaning up the workshop. Each participant filled out a time card and was paid by the hour. (See Photos 1 and 2.)

This project was designed to support itself and was funded by taking prepaid orders for the reindeer. Sample reindeer, "The Reindeer of Hope," were created and displayed at the Hope Center and Eastern Kentucky University where the orders were taken. The money generated by these orders bought supplies and paid the men's salaries. There were so many orders that the men received weekly raises and substantial Christmas bonuses at the end of the workshop. The newspaper and television publicity generated by the workshop boosted the self-esteem of the men as well as the community image of the Hope Center, the University and of occupational therapy. The workshop, supervised by the Level II occupational therapy students with the assistance of Level I students, became a daily afternoon activity. The reindeer workshop lasted for eight weeks, ending with the departure of the Level II students.

PHOTO 1. The Reindeer of Hope, Ready for Delivery

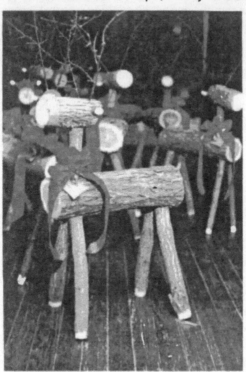

Outcomes of the Occupational Therapy Program

Outcomes were very positive overall. Some outcome measures were formally solicited; some came spontaneously as a result of the program. Staff and clients were given questionnaires to respond to the effectiveness of the occupational therapy program. Seven staff and seven clients responded to this survey.

STAFF RESPONSE

The staff questionnaire consisted of nine questions that could be answered by ranking student or client performance from 1 to 5, the higher rank indicating the more positive response. There were also open-ended questions. See Tables 1 and 2 for summarized responses.

On the ranked questions, staff rated program effectiveness from 4.4 to 4.8, with the professional behaviors of the students receiving slightly higher rat-

PHOTO 2. In the Reindeer Workshop

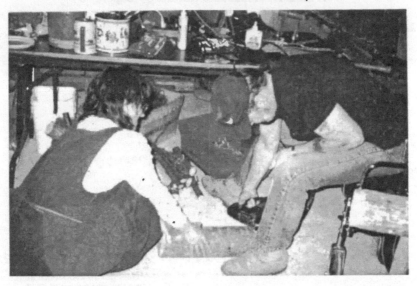

ings than the improvement of the clients. Some primary themes in the narrative responses of the staff include both the amount of and nature of the activities, the improvement in the clients' self-worth, socialization, and the students' concern for the clients. Staff also brought up issues of salary for prospective occupational therapy employees and the need for program development and funding. See Table 2 for summarized staff narrative responses.

CLIENT RESPONSE

While the questions on the staff and client questionnaires addressed the same areas, the client questionnaire had only five questions that could be ranked numerically; the emphasis was on questions that could be answered narratively. Many of the clients had literacy and/or cognitive difficulties, and it was anticipated that they might be more responsive to oral questions. They were offered the choice of speaking to the questions in a group or in individual meetings with the investigator (the first author). Six of the seven respondents preferred individual meetings. One of these chose to give narrative answers to all questions. One respondent filled out the questionnaire independently. Clients' responses were recorded verbatim, and the investigator reviewed all of the respondents' answers with them for accuracy and consent to use them in the program evaluation.

TABLE 1. Ranked and Narrative Responses

Question	Staff Response N = 7	Client Response N = 7
1. Effective interaction	4.8	5
2. Reliable	4.8	5
3. Respectful of others	4.6	5
4. Overall impact of the students	4.6	5
5. More time doing satisfying, productive activities?	4.4	4.8
6. Quality of required, routine activities	4.4	Not asked–included in #7
7. Helped ADLs	4.5	Yes–7 It helped to relearn–1 money management–2 hygiene–3 laundry–3
8. Feel better about themselves/yourself	4.5	Yes–7 They cared how you producted as a person–1 They got us to do more than we thought we could do–1 Reindeer–3
9. Would you want an OT working with you?	4.5	Yes–5, Definitely–2 I don't have the time–1 Time for me to move on–1

The numerical rankings of the clients, 5 for four of the questions and 4.8 for one of the questions, may reflect the clients' attachment to the students. Their narrative responses give a broader and richer picture of their experiences in the program. Predominant themes for the clients included the students appreciating them as individuals and providing productive activities, "not just pencil and paper," as one participant said. All respondents noted improvement in how they felt about themselves and their ability to take care of themselves. The students' attitudes and their care for the men were clearly identified as important factors in the success of this program for the participants.

ADDITIONAL OUTCOMES

Both students expressed that the experience of creating and implementing a program in the community was invaluable to their professional development. Students and faculty found that the learning objectives of this fieldwork in the areas of assessment, treatment planning, treatment, and problem solving were

TABLE 2. Narrative Responses

Question	Staff Response N = 7	Client Response N = 7
10. Best thing about working with OT students	Concern of students for clients–2 Cooking projects–3 Laundry–1 Self-esteem of clients–5 Amount of activity–3 Additional services–3 Increased interaction/social skills–3 Reindeer–3	They learned off of us and we learned off of them–1 Helped me take care of myself–2 Being productive–3 Laundry–2 Cooking–1 What I learned–3 Reindeer–2 Attitude/personalities–4
11. Hardest thing about working with OT students	Not here long enough–2 Not able to spend as much time with them as I want–2 Need to work together to strategize and develop backing to have these programs–1 Not enough time for me to interact with clients–1	Hearing voices while working–1 Saying goodbye–2 Nothing–3 Could communicate better with me sometimes–1
12. What else	Tried to hire an OT–couldn't afford it–1 Excited/appreciative re: results–2 Thank you–4	Got to know one another but didn't fight–1 Nice experience overall–1 Enjoyed myself–1 They care about people and they care deeply–1 Good instructions, especially safety–1 Thank you–3

very effectively met in this situation. The students progressed rapidly through their assignments; they had the needs assessment completed and the screening tool created and in use by week two. The reindeer workshop fulfilled their final project assignment. The only objective they did not meet was participation in outcomes measurement. They were so involved in reindeer production that they felt they could not find the time or energy for this aspect of the experience. This may illustrate some of the difficulties clinicians have with integrating research into practice. In hindsight, the second author became more appreciative of the need for outcomes measurement, as she will submit a federal grant application to support occupational therapy positions and programs as a project to fulfill the requirements for her master's degree.

During the time period of this study, two occupational therapists were interviewed for a position at this facility for the first time. They declined the offered staff position due to the salary. Occupational therapists with a master's degree will be considered for supervisory and administrative positions as they become available. Both authors collaborated with the Hope Center program director to include an occupational therapy position in grant funding for a developing program. The success of the Level II students in the mental health program has allowed expansion of the Level II program to the Recovery Programs at the center.

As this fieldwork and study came to a close, a grant was funded by the Candle Foundation to help support the Eastern Kentucky University Occupational Therapy Program at the Hope Center. This grant will underwrite equipment and supplies for specific projects in all of the programs, including a garden, a health and wellness program and area, and a living skills education program.

DISCUSSION AND CONCLUSIONS

The Hope Center-Eastern Kentucky University collaboration and this Level II fieldwork experience, in particular, continue to demonstrate the positive benefit of occupational therapy with this population. Both client and staff responses validate the efficacy of student involvement in this community setting. While the Hope Center staff had been extremely appreciative of the Level I occupational therapy students (Scaffa, Brownson, & Shordike, 2001), the experience of having Occupational Therapy services available daily, and at a higher level, clarified their understanding of what occupational therapy has to offer. Interestingly, although the reindeer workshop came to dominate the program, both staff and clients recognized the relationship of the ongoing occupational therapy program to the success of the high-profile workshop.

The process of creating and implementing this program reinforced both student and faculty understanding of the uniqueness of occupational therapy and what we can bring to this population. Our discipline's knowledge base, evaluation tools, and training in activity analysis allowed us to work with these clients in ways that maximized their independence and productivity. We understood what these men wanted to do and were capable of, and specifically how to facilitate this. It also further fueled our passion for bringing the work we do into the community.

The participants in the program challenged the student therapists to meet their needs at ever higher levels. This created a reciprocally empowering therapeutic environment, an environment where the clients were eager to express themselves to each other, staff, and the community in general. Once empowered, all of the men in this program were eager to contribute to the community and this study. The authors urge therapists involved in community programs to continue to gather qualitative data, to evaluate outcomes in a way that honors the participation and response of those involved and provides data for evidence-based practice.

REFERENCES

Allen, C.K. (1985). *Occupational therapy for psychiatric diseases: Measurement and management of cognitive disabilities.* Boston: Little, Brown.

Barris, R., Oakley, F., & Kielhofner, G. (1988). The role checklist. In B. Hemphill (Ed.), *Mental health assessment in occupational therapy. An integrative approach to the evaluation process* (pp. 73-91). Thorofare, NJ: Slack.

Barth, T. (1994). Occupational therapy interventions at a shelter for homeless, addicted adults with mental illness. *American Occupational Therapy Association Mental Health Special Interest Section Newsletter, 17* (1), 7-8.

Cnaan, R.A. & Blankertz, L.E. (1993). Serving the dually diagnosed homeless: Program development and interventions. *The Journal of Mental Health Administration, 20,* 100-112.

Drake, M. (1992). Level I fieldwork in a daycare for homeless children. *Occupational Therapy and Psychosocial Dysfunction.* The Haworth Press, Inc., 215-224.

Fischer, P.J. & Breakey, W.R. (1991). The epidemiology of alcohol, drug, and mental disorders among homeless persons. *American Psychologist, 46,* 1115-1128.

Heubner, J. & Tryssenaar, J. (1996). Development of an occupational therapy practice perspective in a homeless shelter: A fieldwork experience. *Canadian Journal of Occupational Therapy, 63,* 24-32.

Interagency Council on the Homeless, U.S. Department of Housing and Urban Development (1994). *Priority: Home! The federal plan to break the cycle of homelessness.* Available from Community Connections, PO Box 7189, Gaithersburg, MD.

Kavanagh, J. & Fares, J. (1995). Using the model of human occupation with homeless mentally ill clients. *British Journal of Occupational Therapy, 58,* 419-422.

Kiesler, C.A. (1991). Homelessness and public policy priorities. *American Psychologist, 46,* 1245-1252.

Kohlman-Thompson, L. (1992). *Kohlman evaluation of living skills.* Rockville, MD: American Occupational Therapy Association.

Kondratas, A. (1991). Ending homelessness. *American Psychologist, 46,* 1226-1231.

Law, M., Baptiste, S., Carswell-Opzoomer, A., McColl, M., Polatajko, H., & Pollack, N. (1994). *Canadian occupational performance measure, 2nd ed.* Toronto: Canadian Association of Occupational Therapists.

Lehman, A.E. & Cordray, D.S. (1993). Prevalence of alcohol, drug, and mental disorders among the homeless: One more time. *Contemporary Drug Problems, 20,* 355-383.

Marks, L. (1997). Homeless program benefits from OT skills. *OT Practice, 7,* 22-23.

Mitchell, H. & Jones, D. (1997). Homelessness: A review of the social policy background and the role of occupational therapy. *British Journal of Occupational Therapy, 60,* 315-319.

National Coalition for the Homeless (1999). *Mental illness and homelessness: Fact sheet #5.* Delmar, NY: National Resource on Homelessness & Mental Illness.

Privott, C.R. (1998). *The fieldwork anthology.* Bethesda, MD: The American Association of Occupational Therapy, Inc.

Rydeen, K., Kautzmann, L., Cowan, M.K., & Benzing, P. (1995). Three faculty facilitated, community-based level I fieldwork programs. *American Journal of Occupational Therapy, 49,* 112-118.

Scaffa, M., Brownson, C., & Shordike, A. (2001: in press) Implications for professional education and research. In M. Scaffa (Ed.), *Occupational Therapy in Community-Based Practice Settings*. Philadelphia: F.A. Davis.

Townsend, E. (1993). Occupational therapy's social vision. *Canadian Journal of Occupational Therapy, 60*, 174-184.

Williams, S. & Bloomer, J. (1987). *The bay area functional performance evaluation (second edition)*. Pequannock, NJ: Maddak, Inc.

Collaborative Learning
Applied to Fieldwork Education

Ellen S. Cohn, ScD, OTR/L, FAOTA
Nancy Robert Dooley, MA, OTR/L
Lynn A. Simmons, MS, OTR/L

SUMMARY. Occupational therapists of the 21st century must be educated to provide intervention within health, education, community, and policy-making areas. Therapists need to solve complex problems, often in collaboration with numerous stakeholders. This article proposes that

---

Ellen S. Cohn is Clinical Associate Professor at Boston University, Sargent College of Health and Rehabilitation Sciences, 635 Commonwealth Avenue, Boston, MA 02215. She was formerly Academic Fieldwork Coordinator at Tufts University-Boston School of Occupational Therapy. While at Tufts, Dr. Cohn taught numerous courses and workshops on collaborative approaches to fieldwork. She has published extensively in the area of fieldwork education and clinical reasoning.

Nancy Robert Dooley is Assistant Professor, Occupational Therapy Assistant Program at New England Institute of Technology, Warwick, RI. She is also a doctoral candidate in the occupational therapy program at New York University. In 1997 she presented a mini-course, "Quantifying the Costs and Benefits of Clinical Education" at the AOTA Annual Conference. She represented Rhode Island at AOTA's Mental Health Partnership Project and currently serves as the mental health special interest section chairperson for her state association.

Lynn A. Simmons is a Senior Occupational Therapist and Student Program Coordinator at Youville Hospital & Rehabilitation Center, Cambridge, MA. She teaches occupational therapy at Bay State College, Boston and Massachusetts Bay Community College, Wellesley. Lynn has been a recipient of the New England Occupational Therapy Education Council's educator award.

[Haworth co-indexing entry note]: "Collaborative Learning Applied to Fieldwork Education." Cohn, Ellen S., Nancy Robert Dooley, and Lynn A. Simmons. Co-published simultaneously in *Occupational Therapy in Health Care* (The Haworth Press, Inc.) Vol. 15, No. 1/2, 2001, pp. 69-83; and: *Education for Occupational Therapy in Health Care: Strategies for the New Millennium* (eds: Patricia Crist, and Marjorie Scaffa) The Haworth Press, Inc., 2001, pp. 69-83. Single or multiple copies of this article are available for a fee from The Haworth Document Delivery Service [1-800-HAWORTH, 9:00 a.m. - 5:00 p.m. (EST). E-mail address: getinfo@haworthpressinc.com].

preparing occupational therapists for current practice requires a fundamental change in our educational beliefs and that a collaborative approach among students and fieldwork educators is most congruent with the interactive environments of current practice. The philosophical principles of collaborative learning are reviewed and practical considerations to apply the principles to Level II fieldwork programs are described. *[Article copies available for a fee from The Haworth Document Delivery Service: 1-800-HAWORTH. E-mail address: <getinfo@haworthpressinc. com> Website: <http://www.HaworthPress.com> © 2001 by The Haworth Press, Inc. All rights reserved.]*

KEYWORDS. Supervision, internships, teaching

The methods educators choose to best prepare students for the 21st century are dependent upon underlying beliefs about learning. Historically, occupational therapists utilized a one-to-one or individualistic model of fieldwork education. Students relied on the fieldwork educator to provide them with correct approaches to practice (Collier & O'Connor, 1998). By passively accepting knowledge from their fieldwork educators, students learned in a competitive atmosphere. Recently, we have shifted away from this "received knowledge" perspective, in which learners were taught isolated skills by experts, to a "process oriented" perspective where students construct and reflect on knowledge related to the context in which it is used (Belenky, Clinchy, Goldberger, & Tarule, 1986; Light & Butterworth, 1993).

The 1998 *Standards for an Accredited Educational Program for the Occupational Therapist* emphasize the value of promoting clinical reasoning and reflective practice during fieldwork experiences. Numerous authors recommend shifting from a technical-skills oriented approach to a process-oriented approach that prepares future practitioners for life-long learning (Cohn, 1989; Cohn & Czycholl, 1991; Eraut, 1994; Mattingly & Fleming, 1994; Rogers, 1983; Royeen, 1995; Parham, 1987; Schon, 1987; West, 1990). This article reviews some of the antecedents to the focus on process, and proposes that a collaborative approach to fieldwork education offers a philosophical framework well-suited to prepare occupational therapists for evolving practice arenas. Practical considerations for applying a collaborative approach in fieldwork settings are also delineated.

A broader view of the learning process requires that we consider the interpersonal and sociocultural context in which future practitioners will be working. Occupational therapists of the 21st century and beyond must be educated to provide services within health, education, community, and policy-making arenas. We now work in environments that emphasize cost containment, realistic functional outcomes, evidence-based practice, and client-centered care. Successful intervention involves a collaborative and mutual process where practitioners and consumers develop intervention plans together (Case-Smith & Wavrek, 1993; Crepeau, 1994; Golin & Ducanis, 1981; Humphry, Gonzalez, & Taylor, 1993; Leff & Walizer, 1992; Neistadt, 1987).

Along with the shift in the health care environment, perspectives on education and learning have also shifted. Rather than placing responsibility for learning on the experts to teach specific skills for a particular situation, responsibility is shifted to the learner to solve the variety of problems confronted in practice. Johnson and Johnson (1991), leading proponents of collaborative learning, delineated principles which highlight contemporary views about learning:

1. Knowledge is constructed, discovered, transformed, and extended by students. The educator creates a setting where students, when given a subject, can explore, question, research, interpret, and solidify the knowledge they feel is important.
2. Students actively construct their own knowledge. Students guided by the educator actively seek out knowledge.
3. Education is a personal transaction among students and between educators and students as they work together.
4. All of the above can only take place within a cooperative context. There is no competition among students to strive to be better than the other. Students take responsibility for each other's learning.

Emerging from these contemporary views of learning is the problem-based learning model (PBL) that emphasizes active student involvement, enabling students to assume the habits of lifelong learning. Using PBL principles, Royeen (1995) designed an occupational therapy curriculum in which students worked in small group tutorials to solve problems. Through PBL, students are enculturated into the process of learning in groups, which simulates the practice environment where therapists work in collaborative teams. More recently, Nolinske and Millis (1999) argued that "lecture-based pedagogical approaches" cannot adequately prepare students in professional and technical occupational therapy programs (p. 31). They advocate strategies to enable students to discover and construct knowledge.

As a result of these shifts in education and health care, interest in applying collaborative learning principles to fieldwork education has blossomed (Bruffee, 1987; Crist, 1993; DeClute & Ladyshewsky, 1993; Horger, 1994;

Ladyshewsky, 1993; Ladyshewsky & Healy, 1990; Stern, 1994; Tiberius & Gaiptman, 1985). Collaborative learning extends beyond putting a group of students together to learn from one fieldwork educator. Collaborative learning is a form of indirect teaching in which the educator states problems and organizes students to solve the problems in peer groups. Interest in collaborative learning is further motivated by our heightened awareness of the critical reasoning demands on therapists. Practitioners must recognize the unique conditions presented by each situation, make careful observations, interpretations, and problem solve with others to develop the best strategies for intervention. Thus, preparing occupational therapists to provide collaborative and wide-ranging services requires a fundamental change in our philosophical beliefs. The focus of this article is to suggest ways in which the philosophical and practical principles of collaborative learning can be applied to occupational therapy fieldwork education.

PHILOSOPHICAL PRINCIPLES OF COLLABORATIVE LEARNING

A compelling theoretical rationale for collaborative learning comes from the Russian psychologist L. S. Vygotsky (Miller, 1993). Emphasizing the role of context and socialization in the creation of knowledge, he claimed that our distinctively human mental functions and accomplishments have their origins in our social relationships. Mental functioning, in his view, is based on the assumption that people learn through group interaction where individuals exchange ideas. This social constructionist view recognizes the possibility of multiple realities because each individual experiences the world from his or her own perspective. Through the group interactive process, individuals learn about the diversity of their individual perspectives and create a unified broad perspective. If we embrace this perspective that knowledge is socially constructed through interaction with people, we can see the value of learning within groups during fieldwork experience.

Vygotsky's community collaboration perspective directly challenges the view of the fieldwork educator as "expert," explicitly telling or showing presumably unknowing students the correct response. Rather than relying solely on the fieldwork educator, learners help each other learn, each according to their abilities. These student collaborations do not exclude the presence or value of role models but shift the role of fieldwork educators to that of conductors "orchestrating" the learning (Bruner, 1996). This role shift does not reduce fieldwork educators' role or authority–rather fieldwork educators encourage students to share the role as self-directed learners and to use each other as primary resources.

Closely linked to Vygotskian community collaboration ideas are the team-work practices derived from social learning theory. These teamwork practices are based upon the principle that students will be more motivated to work hard to help group members when they are working toward a common goal. Thus, the role of the fieldwork educator is to acknowledge a student only when all of the group members succeed in learning. Johnson and Johnson (1990) have identified five basic conditions of a collaborative learning situation:

1. *Positive interdependence*: a recognition by group members that they are linked together in a way that none of them can be successful unless they all are. Students must believe they sink or swim together. Within every cooperative task, students develop mutual learning goals.
2. *Face-to-face interaction*: group members have access to each other's talents and resources and promote each other's success. Students inter-act to help each other accomplish a task.
3. *Individual accountability*: requires each group member to be active, learn, and be able to do the things that they learned in the group. Stu-dents team together so they can subsequently perform at a higher level as individuals. Students are held individually accountable for their share of the work.
4. *Cooperative skills*: need to be encouraged and taught as carefully as the subject matter.
5. *Group processing*: students in cooperative relationships need to process their experiences on an ongoing basis to become more skillful in work-ing as a group. Fieldwork educators need to ensure that members of the group discuss how well they are achieving goals and maintaining effec-tive working relationships. Group members need to identify what is helpful or non-helpful.

These concepts of cooperative relationships define the difference between simply putting students in groups to learn and collaborative learning.

The application of these collaborative learning principles is consistent with our understanding of adult learners (Knowles, 1980). Table 1 highlights the differences between the traditional learning that is based on pedagogical ap-proaches to learning and the collaborative approach that is based upon adult learning principles of androgogy. Adult learners are generally "self-motivated and self-directed learners whose experience orients them to practical issues" (Pecora & Austin, 1987, p. 135). The climate of today's occupational therapy practice arena demands that practitioners be both self-motivated and self-di-rected as they frequently confront new and more complex problems. Thus, we need to prepare future occupational therapists to take control of their learning

TABLE 1. Differences Between Traditional and Collaborative Learning

Traditional	Collaborative
Competitive	Cooperative
FW Educator is expert	FW Educator is co-learner in group
FW Educator is in control of time and response	Group membership shares timing and response
FW Educator in control of content, transfers knowledge to student	Group decides content and sequence, knowledge is jointly constructed and modified by group process
FW Educator establishes learning structure	Group shares responsibility for structure
FW Educator is autonomous	Group is interdependent/share individual roles
Students passive learners	Students active learners
Students work independently, little interaction, impersonal transaction among students	Prolonged interaction, oral rehearsal of material being studied, peer tutoring/learning and general support
Predictable learning objectives	Objectives formed by group

rather than develop dependence upon a fieldwork educator to prescribe what they should learn and when.

Bruffee (1987) argued that "Collaborative learning calls on levels of ingenuity and inventiveness that many students never knew they had. And it teaches interdependence in an increasingly collaborative world that requires greater flexibility and adaptability to change than ever before" (p. 47). Research indicates that if student-student interdependence is structured carefully, students will achieve at a higher level, applying reasoning strategies more frequently, and will be more intrinsically motivated (Johnson & Johnson, 1990). It is these skills that we aim to teach our future occupational therapists.

APPLICATION OF COLLABORATIVE PRINCIPLES TO LEVEL II FIELDWORK

The principles of collaborative learning have been applied in fieldwork education programs at a private psychiatric hospital, a not-for-profit multi-level rehabilitation and long-term care facility for persons with physical disabilities, and a group of community-based adult day programs. Collaborative learning has been used in these settings with student-fieldwork educator ratios of 2:1 and 3:1 for several years and will be described in the following section.

Preparation

Education and preparation are essential for fieldwork educators and students in all fieldwork settings. Students have generally been socialized to approach learning in a competitive manner, and learning with peers in a collaborative manner requires a shift in philosophy. Therefore, prior to developing a collaborative fieldwork education program, everyone involved needs to understand the principles of collaborative learning and make a collective commitment to implementing a collaborative fieldwork education program.

Preparation for implementing a collaborative learning approach to fieldwork education can take many forms and must be tailored to the needs of the occupational therapy department and individuals involved. Revising existing fieldwork programs avoids having to recreate an entirely new program. One way to begin the conversation about collaborative learning is for the staff to review articles articulating the philosophical underpinnings of collaborative learning. The staff could share their impressions of the collaborative approach and brainstorm about how a collaborative approach might work in their particular setting. Such a discussion may serve the additional purpose of identifying any fears, barriers, or misgivings that fieldwork educators may have about giving up their traditional modes of supervision. With these potential barriers identified, steps can be taken to provide additional education or dispel myths.

Conferences and consultation about collaborative learning are frequently available to therapists from local academic programs (Collier & O'Connor, 1998; Joe, 1994) either on-site or off-site. Clinical fieldwork coordinators knowledgeable about collaborative learning may also act as resources for fieldwork educators through regular supervision sessions. At the psychiatric hospital a weekly fieldwork educators meeting was held to examine personal teaching styles, explore educational beliefs, discuss differences between collaborative and traditional learning, address student issues, and provide mutual support. The group analyzed the existing fieldwork program to identify learning activities that could be shifted to a collaborative format. Once the collaborative approach to fieldwork was implemented, the content of the weekly meeting shifted to practical problem solving and discussion of successes and new ideas.

As with any new venture, successes should be nurtured early on. When attempting to replicate the program described here, identification of a few fieldwork educators who are initially enthusiastic about collaborative learning may help generate interest in the model among others (Ladyshewsky & Healey, 1990). Some programs may be particularly conducive to a collaborative approach, perhaps due to the number of clients involved, or the intervention philosophy utilized. For example, at the psychiatric hospital a general therapy unit was selected to use the collaborative approach because it had a large and varied caseload that could easily accommodate two students being added to the occupational therapy team. Furthermore, most of the therapy took place in groups where the student pair could serve as co-leaders, which was already the norm for group leadership.

Prior to the fieldwork experience, students should also be prepared to participate in the collaborative approach to learning. The academic fieldwork coordinator can provide an introduction to the philosophical tenets of collaborative learning and any facility-specific information. The clinical fieldwork coordinator can provide seminars, readings, interviews, or a mailing describing the collaborative approach to fieldwork education. Again, a discussion of assigned articles may be very helpful and may set the stage for collaborative teamwork. In many settings, once the fieldwork experience begins, students attend a weekly peer supervision meeting that is structured and run by the students themselves to facilitate group processing and to maintain effective working relationships.

Forming Student Pairs

Within the realm of collaborative learning, no single approach is recommended for team or pair formation. There are several ways to decide upon student pairs or groupings for collaborative learning. Students may provide background information identifying their prior experiences and learning styles to aid in determining student pairs. Academic fieldwork coordinators sometimes pair students according to academic or personal characteristics (Ladyshewsky & Healey, 1990). This grouping method may not be ideal, however, because it takes the element of choice and control away from the learners at the onset. According to Johnson and Johnson (1991), students should have an active role in the collaborative learning process. When pairs are formed at random, or by the educator, students' individual accountability is diminished. If the student pair encounters difficulty, it may be easier to blame the educator for an unsatisfactory pairing. Another approach to assigning pairs is to ask students to identify desired specialty programs within a large facility.

An innovative approach to pairing students used at the psychiatric hospital is to have students meet the various fieldwork educators and preview the different programs on the first day(s) of the fieldwork experience. Before choosing their collaborative partners, students complete an ice breaker activity together, such as making ice cream together or exploring the grounds of the facility. This shared activity immediately fosters positive interdependence. Allowing students to choose their partners facilitates autonomy and encourages students to take responsibility for their choices from the beginning of the fieldwork experience. Sending students written information in advance regarding the different therapy programs, and asking students to rank their preferences can shorten the decision-making process.

Students from the same academic program may become collaborative pairs; however, students from different academic programs often find an additional richness in their collaboration due to their diverse backgrounds and curricula. At the psychiatric hospital no attempts are made to match students according to academic records or other criteria. The therapists there have found that students with very different academic skills and preparation can form effective collaborative relationships.

Role and Preparation of Fieldwork Educators

In collaborative learning the daily activities and expectations of the fieldwork educator are quite different from the activities and expectations in a traditional one-to-one supervision model. In all fieldwork models, the fieldwork educator can expect to spend time role modeling evaluation, therapy, and other responsibilities in the initial weeks of the learning experience. As students take on more responsibilities, the fieldwork educators usually spend less time modeling for students. When students have a peer to rely on for moral support and clinical reasoning, they tend to use each other to test assumptions and build confidence. The fieldwork educator may spend less time throughout the day shadowing a student, because the students view each other as role models and valid sources of feedback. The fieldwork educator can expect to review documentation or provide feedback on a therapy session only after the students have critiqued each other's work. Thus the fieldwork educator focuses the supervision on refining skills in clinical reasoning, observation, and intervention planning; and students practice the valuable skills of giving and receiving feedback.

An example of a shift in roles for the fieldwork educator comes from the psychiatric hospital where reviewing process at the end of each session was standard practice. Group processing frequently consisted of the student giving a few observations that he or she hoped were "right." The fieldwork educator made comments or asked questions and added observations from a position of power. Using the collaborative approach, the fieldwork educator listens to the students processing the group with each other. He or she then asks questions to further stimulate clinical reasoning or clarify students' observations. The fieldwork educator may add a minor observation or pieces of information, but the students become the authorities on what just occurred in the therapy. All members of the collaborative group are contributing to the collective knowledge base while constructing and extending their own learning.

Ground rules and clearly delineated expectations help reinforce the collaborative learning process. Students are responsible for their own and each other's learning. To promote positive interdependence the students discuss problems and generate multiple options together before seeking advice from the fieldwork educator. In cooperative learning, the approval, feedback, and expectations are provided by peers as well as the fieldwork educator. When students work together toward a common goal, the mutual dependence often motivates them to work hard to help the group, and thereby themselves, succeed. For example, students review each other's progress notes, intervention plans, and other documentation before presenting them to the fieldwork educator. Moreover, students discuss positive and negative points of intervention sessions and client interactions, giving each other critical, complementary, and constructive feedback. The fieldwork educator must respect this process and remind students of the ground rules when they do not use each other as resources first.

Structuring Learning Activities

A critical aspect of collaborative learning is the way the learning activities are structured. As in all fieldwork situations, students should not be expected to perform intervention functions until they are competent to do so. However, an early learning task may be structured to facilitate collaboration. For example, a pair of students could observe the intervention environment and separately write down their observations and questions. The students then share their observations and questions with each other and generate additional questions. This face-to-face interaction produces collective observations that can then be shared with the fieldwork educator to generate a plan for the next step in the learning process. The students are actively creating knowledge and helping to direct their future learning.

In the collaborative approach, the fieldwork educator's client caseload may decrease during the fieldwork experience to a greater extent than in a one-to-one approach. For example, one student may work with four clients at a given time, while the pair may work with six to eight clients. This decrease in caseload may provide the fieldwork educator time for committee work, program development, and special projects. The fieldwork educator should plan to meet with the student pair regularly to process each day's events and plan for future learning activities. These meetings initially may be longer with a student pair than they are with an individual, but they can decrease in frequency over time as the students become accustomed to helping to direct their own learning. The time can also be offset by the fieldwork educator's decreased caseload.

The students often share initial client responsibilities with each other. At the facility for persons with physical disabilities, students maintain a joint caseload and provide co-therapy for five to six weeks. After the sixth week, the students continue to problem solve together while they are gradually assigned an individual caseload. To promote individual accountability, students must demonstrate the skills they learned in their pair by actively designing and implementing intervention without their collaborative partner. The students continue to collaborate on any projects, case studies, or presentations. This collaboration allows students to complete meaningful projects that make a contribution to the occupational therapy department, to clients, or to a research project.

At the psychiatric hospital and the adult day programs, students may begin co-leading groups by the end of the first week of fieldwork. Having students take turns leading different parts of the group fosters individual accountability and active co-leadership. Students may continue to use co-leadership for groups, but they are assigned gradually increasing individual caseloads and individually take responsibility for documentation, intervention planning, and collaboration with the rest of the intervention team. Even when students have individual caseloads, positive interdependence is maintained because students must still seek feedback for clinical reasoning, understanding client interactions, and intervention planning.

In the adult day-program setting, three students participating in a collaborative fieldwork experience worked together to harness their creativity and develop a meaningful program for their facility. Previously, while using a traditional supervision model, student creativity was limited to choosing activities for and leading existing groups. By shifting to a collaborative model, the fieldwork educator enabled the student team to take on more responsibility by presenting them with the problem of designing the entire intervention program for the next month. The students combined their resources to meet the added challenge. The students worked with the program staff and clients and observed their routines to identify barriers and facilitators of occupational performance. Using an occupation-based perspective, the students asked clients about their likes and previous occupations. Based on their new understanding, the students developed new groups to address clients' goals and interests. By sharing group leadership among the three students and the program staff, the students initiated new groups in cooking, self-expression, physical activity, and art. Some groups ran simultaneously and were tailored to people at specific functional levels. At the end of the students' fieldwork experience, program staff observed clients do things they previously thought were impossible such as engaging each other in spontaneous conversation, requesting activities, and experiencing success at occupations they had abandoned. Several clients who had previously engaged in only one repetitive task began to regularly engage in and express enjoyment about the new groups.

Interpersonal Issues

If interpersonal issues threaten the learning process, the fieldwork educator must address concerns with all individuals involved. Eraut (1994) suggests that communication skills are most easily enhanced through practice and feedback with real people in true practice situations. Collaborative learning requires that students communicate with each other effectively and become adept at giving and providing feedback. According to the principles of collaborative learning, one-to-one meetings between fieldwork educators and students can undermine the process and should be avoided. Rather, the fieldwork educator encourages direct discussion of conflicts by the student group or pair and plays a mediating role if necessary. The fieldwork educator must be observant of the group dynamics among students because unspoken conflicts can easily undermine the collaborative learning process. As in any dynamic group situation, confrontation is essential and will usually help the student pair overcome competitiveness or differences in skill or style to attain a productive level of cooperation.

Additionally, both students' progress and areas for improvement are reviewed as a group with the fieldwork educator. This open forum allows critique to come from and be given to each member of the collaborative team, including the fieldwork educator. The fieldwork educator does meet with each student individually at the midterm point of the fieldwork experience to set and review individualized goals, and upon completion of the fieldwork experience to provide an opportunity for more personalized and private feedback.

The following vignette illustrates the five basic tenets of collaborative learning described by Johnson and Johnson (1990). Early in their fieldwork experience, one member of a collaborative student pair, Karen, had difficulty interacting with clients who were hesitant to attend groups or were resistive to intervention. The fieldwork educator and Karen's collaborative student partner, Sarah, noticed unproductive conversations that left Karen angry with some clients. After posing various questions to the student pair, the fieldwork educator explored her hypothesis that Karen's difficulty with these clients may be due to countertransference.

After refreshing the students' memories about countertransference and how it distorts the therapeutic relationship, the fieldwork educator wondered aloud to Karen and Sarah if that might be happening. Seeing Karen's discomfort at this possibility, Sarah discussed how another client produced negative feelings in her. This face to-face interaction and group processing allowed Karen to admit that she always had difficulty with people who did not respond to her initial requests. She was able to name examples from her school and home life in which she became very angry with what others saw as minor resistance or a differing point of view. In the atmosphere of trust created by the open and honest discussion, Sarah described another instance when she noticed Karen interacting in a similar manner. Sarah reflected that she was troubled by the interaction, but did not do anything about what she thought at the time was Karen's problem. The group processing with the fieldwork educator helped Sarah recall that in the collaborative approach students "sink or swim" together. The fieldwork educator made her thought process explicit and modeled the cooperative skills needed for successful collaborative learning. Her open discussion using honest and direct feedback helped the students give and receive feedback.

For the remainder of the affiliation, Karen was individually accountable for reflecting on her interactions with clients and processing them with Sarah. Together the students reported to the fieldwork educator on their progress in building rapport with clients who initially seemed difficult to engage. Each student felt that her colleague had been very instrumental in the learning process. By the end of the fieldwork experience, all three members of the collaborative learning team felt that they had grown personally and professionally and improved their abilities to give and accept feedback. This vignette illustrates how potential barriers can be turned into assets in a collaborative learning situation. Our experience with collaborative supervision has been positive and empowering for students and fieldwork educators.

CONCLUSION

The 1997 American Occupational Therapy Association Philosophy of Education states, "Occupational therapy education is grounded in a shared belief that humans are complex beings engaged in an interactive process of continuous adaptation and growth influenced by their physical, social, and cultural environments" (p. 867). This philosophy is consistent with the collaborative learning ideal that emphasizes the role of context and socialization in the creation of knowledge. The experiences presented in this article demonstrate that collaborative learning can be applied in settings using either individual or group approach to intervention and in both institutional and community-based settings.

The genuine applications of collaborative learning move beyond having one fieldwork educator supervise two students simultaneously. When the principles of positive interdependence, face-to-face interaction, individual accountability, cooperative skills and group processing are built into the structure of the fieldwork learning experiences, students learn to problem solve together and develop creative intervention plans. Our experiences have convinced us that a collaborative approach to preparing future practitioners offers students a model for life-long learning most congruent with the interactive environments of current practice.

REFERENCES

Accreditation Council for Occupational Therapy Education of the American Occupational Therapy Association (1998). *Standards for an accredited educational program for the occupational therapist.* Bethesda, MD: American Occupational Therapy Association.

American Occupational Therapy Association (1997). Philosophy of education. *American Journal of Occupational Therapy, 51*, 867.

Belenky, M.F., Clinchy, B.M., Goldberger, N.R., & Tarule, J.M. (1986). *Women's ways of knowing.* New York: Basic Books.

Bruffee, K.A. (1987). The art of collaborative learning: Making the most of knowledgeable peers. *Change, 19,* 671-674.

Bruner, J. (1996). *The culture of education.* Cambridge, MA: Harvard University Press.

Case-Smith, J. & Wavrek, B. (1993). Models of service delivery and team interaction. In J. Case-Smith (Ed.), *Pediatric occupational therapy and early intervention* (pp. 127-159).

Cohn, E.S. (1989). Fieldwork education: Shaping a foundation for clinical reasoning. *American Journal of Occupational Therapy, 43,* 240-244.

Cohn, E.S. & Czycholl, C.M. (1991). Facilitating a foundation for clinical reasoning. In E.B. Crepeau & T. LaGarde (Eds.), *Self-paced instruction for clinical education and supervision: An instructional guide* (pp. 159-182). Rockville, MD: American Occupational Therapy Association.

Collier, G.A. & O'Connor, L. (1998, April). Collaborative supervision, real-life skills. *OT Practice,* pp. 46-48.

Crepeau, E.B. (1994). Uneasy alliances: Belief and action on a geropsychiatric team. (Doctoral dissertation, University of New Hampshire, 1994). *Dissertation Abstracts International,* 9506410.

Crist, P.A. (1993, January 13). Issues in fieldwork education. *Advance for Occupational Therapists,* 2.

DeClute, J. & Ladyshewsky, R. (1993). Enhancing clinical competence using a collaborative clinical education model. *Physical Therapy, 73,* 683-697.

Eraut, M. (1994). *Developing professional knowledge and competence*. Washington, DC: Falmer.

Golin, A.K. & Ducanis, A.J. (1981). *The interdisciplinary team: A Handbook for the Education of Exceptional Children*. Bethesda, MD: Aspen.

Horger, M.M. (1994). Cooperative learning and occupational therapy: A natural combination. *Education Special Interest Section Newsletter, 17*, 1-2.

Humphry, R., Gonzalez, S., & Taylor, E. (1993). Family involvement in practice: Issues and attitudes. *American Journal of Occupational Therapy, 47*, 587-593.

Joe, B. (1994, October 13). Are two heads better than one? *OT Week*, 18-19.

Johnson, D.W. & Johnson, R.T. (1990). *Learning together and alone: Cooperative, competitive and individualistic learning*. Boston: Allyn and Bacon.

Knowles, M. (1980). *The modern practice of adult education*. New York: Association Press.

Ladyshewsky, R. (1993). Clinical teaching and the 2:1 student to clinical instructor ratio. *Journal of Physical Therapy Education, 7*, 31-35.

Ladyshewsky, R. & Healey, E. (1990). *The 2:1 teaching model in clinical education: A manual for clinical instructors*. Toronto: University of Toronto, Department of Rehabilitation Medicine.

Leff, P.T. & Walizer, E.H. (1992). *Building the healing partnership: Parents, professionals & children with chronic illnesses and disabilities*. Cambridge, MA: Brookline Books.

Light, P. & Butterworth, G. (1993). *Context and cognition: Ways of learning and knowing*. Hillsdale, NJ: Lawerence Erlbaum Assoc.

Mattingly, C. & Fleming, M.H. (1994). *Clinical reasoning: Forms of inquiry in therapeutic practice*. Philadelphia: F.A. Davis Co.

Miller, P.H. (1992). *Theories of developmental psychology* (3rd ed.). New York: W.H. Freeman and Company.

Neistadt, M.E. (1987). An occupational therapy program for adults with developmental disabilities. *American Journal of Occupational Therapy, 41*, 433-438.

Nolinske, T. & Millis, B. (1999). Cooperative learning as an approach to pedagogy. *American Journal of Occupational Therapy, 53*, 31-43.

Parham, D. (1987). Toward professionalism: The reflective therapist. *American Journal of Occupational Therapy, 41*, 555-561.

Pecora, P. & Austin, M. (1987). *Managing human services personnel*. Newbury, CA: Sage.

Rogers, J.C. (1983). Eleanor Clarke Slagle Lectureship-1983; Clinical reasoning: The ethics, science, and art. *American Journal of Occupational Therapy, 37*, 601-616.

Royeen, C.B. (1995). A problem-based learning curriculum for occupational therapy education. *American Journal of Occupational Therapy, 49*, 338-346.

Schon, D. (1987). *Educating the reflective practitioner: How professionals think in action*. New York: Basic Books.

Stern, K. (1994). Cooperative learning: Increasing achievement in the classroom. *Education Special Interest Section Newsletter, 17*, 3-4.

Tiberius, R. & Gaiptman, B. (1985). Supervisor-student ratio: 1:1 versus 1:2. *Canadian Journal of Occupational Therapy, 52*, 179-183.

West, W.L. (1990). Nationally speaking—perspective on the past and future, Part 2. *American Journal of Occupational Therapy, 44*, 9-10.

Group Co-Leadership
by Occupational Therapy Students
in Community Centers:
Learning Transitional Roles

Mary V. Donohue, PhD, OT, FAOTA

SUMMARY. The experience of contact with community populations and settings at the beginning of fieldwork is essential in expanding the dimensions of non-traditional skills and roles for occupational therapy students. This article describes an initial fieldwork experience which builds on an occupational therapy group process course to enable students to supplement a community-based program with activities designed to meet a need of their group at the appropriate level of group interaction. Pairs of students select a receptive community site prior to the beginning of fieldwork to open dialog with the center's coordinator regarding performance areas, components, or contexts needed by the group. Working to assess the current programmatic offerings and desires of the participants for new activities and planning activities in collaboration with local staff, the students propose to conduct a series of five sessions addressing a theme desired or needed by the group. Upon immersion in the site's program, students are able to provide an in-depth

---

Mary V. Donohue is Clinical Associate Professor, Department of Occupational Therapy, New York University, 35 West Fourth Street, New York, NY 10012 (E-mail: MVD1@nyu.edu).

The author thanks Aliza Reshotko for her review of this article.

[Haworth co-indexing entry note]: "Group Co-Leadership by Occupational Therapy Students in Community Centers: Learning Transitional Roles." Donohue, Mary V. Co-published simultaneously in *Occupational Therapy in Health Care* (The Haworth Press, Inc.) Vol. 15, No. 1/2, 2001, pp. 85-98; and: *Education for Occupational Therapy in Health Care: Strategies for the New Millennium* (eds: Patricia Crist, and Marjorie Scaffa) The Haworth Press, Inc., 2001, pp. 85-98. Single or multiple copies of this article are available for a fee from The Haworth Document Delivery Service [1-800-HAWORTH, 9:00 a.m. - 5:00 p.m. (EST). E-mail address: getinfo@haworthpressinc.com].

assessment of the community group's psychosocial skill needs using the Group Level of Function Profile (Donohue, 2000). *[Article copies available for a fee from The Haworth Document Delivery Service: 1-800-HAWORTH. E-mail address: <getinfo@haworthpressinc.com> Website: <http://www.HaworthPress. com> © 2001 by The Haworth Press, Inc. All rights reserved.]*

KEYWORDS. Cooperative learning, experiential learning, leadership styles

Practicing group leadership roles through peer learning strategies in the community provides an opportunity to expand on the cooperative learning of the classroom. The experiential learning of an activity group process course designed along the lines of occupational therapy principles (Borg & Bruce, 1991; Cole, 1998; Howe & Schwartzberg, 1995; Posthuma, 1999) provides the opportunity for occupational therapy students to become part of an effective group. The effective group, as outlined by Johnson and Johnson (2000), describes a group with many of the characteristics of the curative factors of groups. These group capacities were partly derived from occupational therapy groups: cooperative goals, clear communication, shared leadership, joint problem-solving, a climate of support, norms of responsibility, trust, cohesion, along with the open negotiation of conflicts. In terms defined by Mosey (1986), these traits describe people operating at the level of a cooperative group and a mature group (Borg & Bruce, 1991; Cole, 1998; Howe & Schwartzberg, 1995; Posthuma, 1999).

In the academic activity group process course, general principles of leadership theory are presented regarding leadership style (Johnson & Johnson, 2000; Lewin, Lippit, & White, 1939; Bonner, 1959), describing the charismatic, autocratic, bureaucratic, democratic, and laissez-faire style leadership methods. Other models of leadership are also taught providing varying perspectives, such as the telling, selling, participating, and delegating schema (Borg & Bruce, 1991; Tannenbaum & Schmidt, 1985). Contingency theory of situational leadership style, which is dependent on the task and the level of group ability (Fiedler, 1967), is appropriate for the framework of occupational therapy group intervention. Occupational therapists are prepared to assess the difficulty of the task and the maturity of the group's participants, employing several leadership styles appropriate across a session, day, or week. In an occupational therapy group, giving instruction around a task, allowing for periods of creativity, and encouraging a collaborative discussion of the interaction during the group demand a variety of styles from the leader, perhaps even within one group session (Posthuma, 1999). The intersection of some models, such as that of Tannenbaum and Schmidt with that of Mosey's gradual developmental group levels, gives the students choices in selecting leadership style models (Perkins, 1992). In the lab groups, identification of and assumption of the Bales' goal achievement tasks and maintenance roles (1950) in a purposeful manner also provide a variety of avenues of influencing groups and individuals.

CO-LEADERSHIP THEORY, TRAINING, AND EXPERIENCE IN THE ACADEMIC COURSE: ACTIVITY GROUP PROCESS

For the students to provide a productive learning and/or therapeutic group, their work must be preceded by the structured development of an effective group of their own (Johnson & Johnson, 2000). The academic course in occupational therapy group process was designed as an integral part of the entry-level curriculum at New York University and provides a model of co-leadership as it is presented by professors in the lecture. Students have opportunity in their labs to demonstrate and practice both individual and co-leadership of groups during this fourteen-week academic course.

Using principles of co-leadership presented by Crowther (1991), Scott (2000), and Wilson and Kneisel (1992), students are presented with an academic lab setting encouraging interactional communication for more effective functioning as partners. Issues of attraction, power, and style of the leaders are discussed in lecture and lab. For example, leader partners are coached to sit apart in the group so as to spread out the power foci of leadership. They are presented with the concepts of both symmetrical and complementary types of partnerships (Crowther, 1991). In the symmetrical relationship the partners balance each other in leadership of most activities and topics, whereas in the complementary relationship, partners highlight aspects of supplementary strengths which they bring to the partnership, permitting each to exhibit differing roles. In both styles, discussing the approximate "percentage" of frequency of leadership expressed by each member of the pair in a balanced co-therapy dyad is essential. During the academic course of occupational therapy group process and the seminar for the community-centered fieldwork, co-leaders are cautioned not to present a partnership of less than a 60:40 ratio of balance of leadership effort on the part of each student. Advantages and disadvantages of co-leadership are presented in lecture (Crowther, 1991; Johnson & Johnson, 2000).

To encourage partner interaction, a handout of Questions from the Group Co-leader's Inventory (Crowther, 1991) is provided in lecture. This questionnaire examines co-leader style, behavior patterns, roles, norms, goals, and ethics. Discussion of its issues in lecture, lab, and between student partners provides a cooperative learning environment for both the academic and fieldwork courses.

A major element presented in the academic course is the identification of the needs of the group of students in each lab as part of planning the co-leadership role sessions for the process course presentations. The group as a whole cooperates to find consensus for a need of most group members, such as stress reduction, assertiveness training, or wellness. The satisfaction of this need then becomes a joint group goal. At this point the lab members collaboratively plan the sequence of sessions for the topical series. Every effort is made to provide a variety of activities within the series, so that a range of activities, such as movement, reading brief articles, food preparation, relevant crafts, discussion and feedback, can be incorporated in the co-leadership series. Partners within the lab group are selected, and the session sub-topics presented by each pair are chosen based on their knowledge, perspective, and experience. Finally, partners begin their collaborative work of planning their lab group co-leadership activity designed to meet the needs of their group. They research their sub-topic in books and on the Internet, in addition to consulting with lab group faculty regarding their projected intervention activities which they propose in order to achieve their group's goal. This cooperative learning style (Johnson & Johnson, 2000) in the academic group course is a prototype of the process the students are expected to pursue in the first fieldwork and seminar course in community centers as paired leaders the following summer.

GROUP CO-LEADERSHIP
IN COMMUNITY FIELDWORK CENTERS:
FIELDWORK I

In recent years, the needs of society and the changing definition of health as it expands into the community have been emphasized by occupational therapists in listening to consumer needs (Baum & Law, 1998). The theory of service of occupational therapy includes a gradually expanding focus on client-centered needs in community-based rehabilitation (CBR, McColl, 1998). While there are a number of models for setting up non-traditional community practice roles for students to enter the non-clinical arena, which have been presented in the occupational therapy literature (Brownson, 1998; Fleming, Christenson, Franz, & Letourneau, 1996; Drake, 1992; Scott, 1999; Vanier & Hebert, 1995), this fieldwork with group seminars provides an alternative approach, linking fieldwork with the educational process (Opacich, 1995). Likewise, the suggestion of giving serious consideration to fieldwork placements not supervised by occupational therapists is being increasingly valued (Hamlin, MacRae, & DeBrakeleer, 1995).

The co-leadership method is both a service to the community and a cooperative learning experience for the students. It provides the students with an opportunity to offer leadership at the site in two ways. Students are encouraged to work both collaboratively with each other and with the center, as well as independently to introduce creative ideas and occupational therapy approaches through their leadership practice (Scott, 2000). An example of a distinct occupational therapy group approach consists of processing the group's issues with the group at its conclusion to enable a reflective as well as a concrete result from the group meeting. Students are guided to respectfully assess group needs in the community site conjointly with supervisors and staff, enabling students to provide leadership for new directions of activity need satisfaction and innovation to the program at the center (Drake, 1992). Simultaneously, the partners plan the organization and tone of their group, providing leadership to the consumers in keeping with their highest level of group interaction. This is carried out as the students immerse themselves in their group and evaluate in detail the spectrum of the group's potential for developmental progress through parallel, project, egocentric cooperative, cooperative, and mature groups (Donohue, 1999; Mosey, 1986). Empowerment of students as competent group co-leaders in their new role is emphasized.

In weekly seminars during the community fieldwork experience, students are coached to enable groups to function at their highest potential of interaction, initiative, and responsibility. For example, questions to students co-leading adult groups guide them to ask themselves: "Could this group operate through mutual group leadership on their own after the five-week series by using cooperative level and mature level group skills?" In other words, "Could the group continue the activity intervention on their own?" The student partners are encouraged to prepare the group to become a mutual leadership group, if the group has the potential to function in this manner.

In describing several types of curriculum design used with the student partners in the fieldwork course, four types will be highlighted: (1) the procedural process of student co-leaders setting up community sites for fieldwork, (2) the pragmatic considerations of working with the limitations of specific populations, (3) the conditional basis for leadership styles contingent on the activities needed to supplement the community group's program, and (4) interactive reasoning in seminars and in consultation with on-site teachers, principals, and directors of centers and schools. These curriculum designs will be noted in titles of some of the following sections.

PROCESS OF SETTING UP COMMUNITY SITE FIELDWORK: PROCEDURAL CURRICULUM DESIGN

Three months prior to their first fieldwork, students contact community centers for their summer group co-leadership role experience. The student partners frequently live near each other or select central sites to explore together. A loose-leaf binder of information regarding previously selected community settings available in the occupational therapy department serves as a guide in selecting a location with a population feasible for them to work with in ongoing groups. Table 1 presents a timeline of steps in the preparation for community-based fieldwork. The student pairs then call the center for an appointment to meet the director of the center or principal of the school. When they meet for their appointment, the students discuss the needs of the group or ask about an area in the program that may need supplementation.

Later the students pay a more in-depth visit to their selected site, asking to observe groups briefly, inquiring about whether needs exist, and requesting to know which activities the group enjoys. Examining strengths of the group, as well as areas of interest and need, the student partners assess what the performance areas, performance components, and performance contexts are that relate to these needs. Writing up a mini-assessment outline of the areas of need, students suggest a tentative series of activities to the director, principal, or teacher in their second, more formal meeting. They ask for feedback and guid-

TABLE 1. Timeline of Preparation for and Involvement in Community-Based Fieldwork

Calendar	Presentations and Assignments
Fall Semester	Occupational Therapy Group Process–Academic course–with labs
	Practice/training in labs in leadership and co-leadership skills
Spring Semester	Orientation meeting for community fieldwork preparation
	Select a partner
	Process of search for a site by student partners
February	Three preliminary sites suggested on form
March	Preliminary Assessment of Group Member's Activity Needs–form with signature of principal or director from site decided upon
Summer Semester	Week one–Begin community fieldwork–orientation and planning
May	Week two–Protocol of sequence of five sessions
June	Week three–Orientation/training for Group Level of Function Profile
	Week four–Group Needs Assessment
	Week five–Work on posters with photographs of group member
	Week six–Luncheon with supervisors with posters on display

ance in reviewing their selection with their future supervisor. This process immerses them in experiencing the role of relating to community organizations or systems. Some centers are very directive in indicating what they believe the needs of their groups might be, in contrast to others who leave the selection up to the students. While welcoming the students, some centers are skeptical about group members' interest in anything new. Whether this represents staff who are "stuck" or inflexible group members, most often the staff and groups are pleasantly surprised by the response to the student co-leaders' excitement for new activities and a new group format.

Moving assertively into the community to search for locations which welcome student assistance takes leadership qualities. The students support each other in this endeavor, discuss strategies, and evaluate needs of the groups in the center, as well as scrutinize their own leadership skills, roles, strengths, and methods. Several years ago two students wished to do their community fieldwork at a particular "Y" well-known for its extensive program with almost every imaginable offering. The director told the student partners that there was nothing they could offer as an activity that the center did not already have. Students have been told in the orientation that if a center they approach does not seem interested in what they have to offer, not to force the issue or themselves on the center; that many centers would be delighted to have them; and that they should go where they are appreciated. The students suggested that they believed that the seniors at the center could use help in learning how to e-mail their grandchildren. Finally, with this suggestion, they were accepted at the "Y." The activity was so popular that fifty people signed up, and the "Y" is now continuing to offer this program.

POPULATIONS AT FIELDWORK SITES REQUIRE PRAGMATIC CURRICULUM DESIGN

Students are directed to select non-traditional sites in the community serving relatively well people. Their population selections usually are groups of typically developing, non-deprived preschool children and non-disabled groups at senior centers. Other choices of groups have included groups in supported living centers and nursing homes, homeless seniors at a residence, Ys, elementary school classes, headstart and settlement preschool groups, battered women in a secure safe house, independent disabled people who are homeless, diagnostic and treatment senior centers, and a teen after-school center. Some sites are affiliated with religious groups, which sometimes become a prominent cultural influence in a center's group life, and in other instances, culture is not a strong element of influence.

One after-school program for adolescents in a beachside community with kids who otherwise would have become latch-key kids, or groups hanging out at a school playground, was organized around a seaside theme. The students assessed that the adolescents were motivated to learn about beach wildlife, needed to learn how to work together, could use funding for their activities, and were unsure about their social sex roles and meaningful relationships. The students' leadership led the adolescents to learn how to fish, study seashore life, raise money for party activities, develop teamwork, and learn how to enjoy the beach environment in a safe manner. The teens were initially relatively directionless and felt uncared for. The student partners gently and enthusiastically shaped them into a group with a more healthy focus.

Another memorable young adolescent group had a strong interest in playground basketball, but had always just hung out, shooting baskets. The partners who worked with them helped them through basketball to see their strengths as a team, as well as their individual strengths to contribute to the team, resulting in their readiness to join a competitive league. The students led this "lost" population into an experience and recognition of their sports abilities.

Some aspects of a group's interaction, or lack of interaction, are not always immediately apparent. In one group of seniors, a husband and wife revealed after some time that they were survivors of the holocaust, which made them wish initially to keep this information secret from their reminiscence group. They did not want to focus the group on negative memories. In another location surprising information that emerged about an apparently average group of preschoolers in a relatively upscale neighborhood was that a number of their parents were very successful "high-end" drug dealers. At another site, an unanticipated behavior which influenced the climate of the group for the members of an affluent supported-living program was a demeaning staff person who humiliated members by encouraging them to kiss each other. At another location, authoritarian or narrow-minded teachers serving as on-site supervisors affected the environment of the group of preschool children and their group interactive behaviors in a negative manner.

ACTIVITIES NEEDED
TO SUPPLEMENT COMMUNITY SITE PROGRAM:
ASSESSMENT OF CONDITIONAL ISSUES
IN CURRICULUM DESIGN

About three months prior to entering their community site, the students are required to observe a potential group of participants at their future center site, meet with the supervisor to discuss the needs of the members and the program, and do a Preliminary Assessment of the Group Members' Activity Needs. This includes indicating Performance Areas of activities of daily living, work, and productive activities or play/leisure activities; Performance Components: sensori-motor, cognitive, or psychosocial components that flow from the Performance Area needs cited; and the Performance Contexts: temporal and environmental aspects that press on the people and the center or school. Lastly, in this preliminary assessment the students are asked to indicate possible group activities that could meet or alleviate the needs indicated above. The student partners write up this assessment together, and then meet with the center's supervisor or the school's director to review the assessment and tentative plan. The supervisor is asked to sign the preliminary assessment before the student submits it to faculty six weeks prior to this fieldwork course.

Children's Activities. Some preschools have a philosophy of total free play, so the student partners together assessed that the children needed some structured activity with organized steps planned in advance. Other preschoolers have been over-organized in their activities and were found to be able to explore creatively with art, music, and imaginative play. Programs with little movement for the children were offered physical activities to experience and encourage movement. Older children in an after-school program were asked what activities they had an interest in pursuing that appealed to them individually and collectively.

Student partners in several preschools in economically deprived areas where there was no structure to the activities noted that whole groups of five-year-olds did not know the letters of their name or of the alphabet, nor did they know numbers. Students were advised in seminar that while they could not take on a whole reading readiness program, because that was not their agreed-upon objective, they could introduce alphabet and number songs and games, interspersed with their previously planned activities.

Adult Activities. Activities frequently requested for seniors at community centers, supported-living residences, and nursing homes include those promoting the goals of socialization, self-esteem, and integration of earlier life stages; activities such as reminiscence groups, current events, movement to music, making greeting cards, framing and mounting photographs, horticulture, impersonating favorite actors and actresses, social/cultural based activities, relaxation and stress reduction activities, cooking for fun, creative writing, crafts activities, and role playing assertive scenarios.

With some senior groups, their activities seem to have been selected for them, so that there was little space for creativity around the selection of activities for group sessions or within sessions around the activity's dimensions. In such instances, the students first modeled creativity suggestions for the senior group; then they offered the group more scope in its choices.

One pair of student partners found that the seniors' reminiscences emerged strongly around actors and actresses whom they had idolized in the early days of movies. Describing why they liked certain actors or actresses as role models, writing scripts for themselves to play typical scenarios selected by them, writing a play together with all their favorite characters included, and, at the end of the series, participating in an academy award night were exciting activities for these seniors.

Session Sequence Protocols

A protocol of session plans for the five sessions the student partners will present over the six weeks is completed by them by the second week on-site during the summer session. It is recommended that the students review this protocol with their principal or director before submitting it to the occupational therapy faculty. The protocols require the students to review the needs/goals of their group in person through observing the group or collecting information from a one-page group survey indicating what the group would need and enjoy. The protocol outline guides the students to indicate their selection of activities designed to meet the needs, goals, or interests of the group members. The matching of the need/goal with specific activities is sometimes challenging for students and becomes a point of discussion in the weekly seminars. Feedback around inappropriate linkages of needs/goals/interests and activities selected by the students is immediately provided so as to enable students to choose activity interventions that meet the group's needs/goals/interests.

FOURFOLD ASSESSMENT OF GROUP BY CO-LEADERSHIP PARTNERS: INTERACTIVE REASONING CURRICULUM DESIGN

Beginning with the initial assessment three months prior to the community fieldwork, jointly evaluating the needs, goals, and strengths of the group with the supervisor and each other, the co-leader student partners assess their group four times (see Table 1). At the outset of the formation of the group in the community, the co-leader partners review the needs, goals, and interests of the group and link these to activities that are facilitating the interventions that the members need. The second assessment of the group takes place just prior to the on-site work by forming these links into a session sequence protocol plan for the five sessions of the series at each site.

The third assessment is an in-depth evaluation that the partners write while on-site, scrutinizing the profile of the members of the group, the population the group represents, and the performance area, components and context unique to their group. Within this assessment the partners choose a group type that they evaluate as fitting the membership to organize their perception of the group's needs/goals and interests: developmental, topical, reference, task, thematic, developmental, and instrumental (Mosey, 1986). The concluding portion of this assessment consists of a section asking the partners to jointly examine the thought processes which influenced their decision-making, writing their step-by-step "clinical" analysis and planning process. These thought processes are requested to enable the partners to reflect back on their perspectives on the group, hopefully coming to better understand their own reasoning. Fourthly, the students collaborate on carrying out an assessment using the Group Level of Function Profile (Donohue, 2000) to ascertain the range of their group's capacity for interaction as Parallel, Project, Egocentric Cooperative, Cooperative, and Mature levels of function examining the group's communication, norms, roles, cooperation, activity behavior, power, and attraction in the group.

Seminars: Interactive Reasoning Curriculum Design

The weekly seminars are approached as group supervision (Crepeau & LaGarde, 1991; Frum & Opacich, 1987; Donohue & McCreedy, 1992). Students describe and discuss both problems and successes. Clinical reasoning is undertaken as group problem-solving for the variety of situations which arise (Mitchell & Kampfe, 1990). Students are curious to hear what is happening at other sites. In the seminar of week two, students are subdivided into two groups for those at sites with seniors and those with preschool children to focus on these two specialty areas separately for one seminar.

The range of cultures, socioeconomic status, and organizational philosophies in the tri-state area is far-reaching, requiring a variety of leadership styles of the student partners. Sites can range from educationally deprived to enriched. Varying approaches are discussed depending on the age, cultural perspective, economic need, and interests of the group members. An array of leadership styles are modeled and discussed in the seminars, depending on the structure or topic of the day and the time allotment. Various coping strategies that the students might employ are considered and weighed as the cultural scenarios are assessed (Mitchell & Kampfe, 1990).

The partners are encouraged not only to use the seminar for support around difficult situations, groups, or supervisors, but also to encourage each other by sharing the positive responses to their leadership and the activities they facilitate in the spirit of a positive focus (Csikszentmihalyi & Seligman, 2000). The seminar helps the partners sort out typical day-to-day problems, and situations requiring a private meeting with a supervisor, teacher, or director. When needed, it is recommended that partners seek on-site supervision, as in the case of the students whose reminiscence group included a couple who had survived the holocaust. The resulting alliance of students, director and social worker on-site at the senior center brought about a permanent establishment of the reminiscence group led by a retired psychologist, a programmatic addition facilitated by student co-leadership.

In one instance students who observed an inappropriate, humiliating, and semi-sexual interaction between an aide and some seniors requested a special meeting with a supervisor. This resulted not only in the remediation of the situation, but also in two of the students' supervisors attending our luncheon, lauding the work of the student partners–their enthusiastic groupwork and their assertive intervention. Group confidentiality in the seminars is stressed, and delicate situations are followed up by individual meetings with the seminar faculty.

The Group Level of Function Profile

This Profile (Donohue, 2000) assists the students in appraising the range of functional levels of which their group is capable. Its use operationalizes the observational perceptions of student partners of their groups. It enables them to identify the skills needed to perform at a given level of function in a group. It further assists those working with seniors to determine whether the group has the capacity to carry on the activities initiated by the students on their own in the future after the departure of the student partners: specifically, can the group function at a cooperative and mature level in order to provide the skills of both task and maintenance roles needed to continue the program through mutual group leadership? Again, in the perspective of positive psychology, the students are encouraged to help the group emphasize their strengths (Csikszentmihalyi & Seligman, 2000). Data gathered from these observations has been incorporated into the research projects of some students in the following semester.

CONCLUSION

Student partners are each given separate grades by their fieldwork supervisors. This fieldwork grade comprises fifty percent of their final grade, so that while written assignments are worked on jointly, the student's final grade also can be different from his/her partner's final grade.

In one assignment students are asked to take photographs of their group in action and make up a poster of their activities to enable the seminar faculty to obtain a glimpse of what occurred at the center. As we well know, pictures are worth a thousand words, and these photographs set up an opportunity for students to proudly display and talk about their groups and their activity series at an end-of-course luncheon to which their supervisors are invited. The exchanges at the luncheon are warm and satisfying, a good beginning tone for the opening of the fieldwork series.

The photographs of one poster still easily come to mind–a group of seniors putting on a fashion show with their favorite night-out-on-the-town gear, clothes they have sewn themselves, or stoles they crocheted, and special attire they would wear to a wedding. There were one or two people in wheelchairs moving down the "runway" to music, decked out in fashionable dress . . .

REFERENCES

Baum, C. & Law, M. (1998). Nationally speaking–Community health: A responsibility, an opportunity, and a fit for occupational therapy. *American Journal of Occupational Therapy, 52,* 7-10.

Borg, B. & Bruce, M. A. (1991). *The group system. The therapeutic activity group in occupational therapy.* Thorofare, NJ: Slack, Inc.

Brownson, C. A. (1998). Funding community practice: Stage 1. *American Journal of Occupational Therapy, 52,* 60-64.

Cole, M. (1998). *Group dynamics in occupational therapy* (2nd ed.) Thorofare, NJ: Slack, Inc.

Crepeau, E. B. & LaGarde, T. (Eds.). (1991). *Self-paced instruction for clinical educational supervision* (SPICES). Rockville, MD: AOTA.

Crowther, D. (1991). Cotherapists: Learning to work together. *Perspectives in Psychiatric Care, 27,* 18-25.

Csikszentmihalyi, M. & Seligman, M. E. P. (2000). Positive psychology: An introduction. *American Psychologist, 55,* 5-14.

Donohue, M. V. (1999). Theoretical bases of Mosey's group interaction skills. *Occupational Therapy International, 6,* 35-51.

Donohue, M. V. (2000). Group Level of Function Profile. Unpublished assessment tool.

Drake, M. (1992). Level I fieldwork in a daycare for homeless children. *Occupational Therapy in Mental Health, 8,* 215-224.

Fiedler, F. E. (1967). *A theory of leadership effectiveness.* New York: McGraw-Hill.

Fleming, J. D., Christenson, J., Franz, D. & Letourneau, L. (1996). A fieldwork model for non-traditional community practice. *Occupational Therapy in Health Care, 10,* 15-35.

Frum, D. C. & Opacich, K. J. (1987). *Supervision: Development of therapeutic competence.* Rockville, MD: American Occupational Therapy Association and Rush University.

Hamlin, R. B., MacRae, N. & DeBrakeleer, B. (1995). Will the Opacich fieldwork model work? *American Journal of Occupational Therapy, 49,* 165-167.

Howe, M. & Schwartzberg, S. (1995). *A functional approach to group work* (2nd ed). Philadelphia: Lippincott.

Johnson, D. W. & Johnson, F. P. (2000). *Joining together. Group theory and group skills.* Boston: Allyn & Bacon.

Lewin, K., Lippitt, R. & White, R. K. (1939). Patterns of aggressive behavior in experimentally created "social climates." *Journal of Social Psychology, 10,* 271-299.

McColl, M. A. (1998). What do we need to know to practice occupational therapy in the community? *American Journal of Occupational Therapy, 52,* 11-18.

Mitchell, M. M. & Kampfe, C. M. (1990). Coping strategies used by occupational therapy students during fieldwork: An exploratory study. *The American Journal of Occupational Therapy, 44,* 543-550.

Mosey, A. C. (1986). *Psychosocial components of occupational therapy.* New York: Raven.

Opacich, K. J. (1995). Is an educational philosophy missing from the fieldwork solution? *The American Journal of Occupational Therapy, 49,* 160-164.

Perkins, V. J. (1992). A model for selecting leadership styles. *Occupational Therapy in Health Care, 8,* 225-237.

Posthuma, B. (1999). *Small groups in counseling and therapy. Process and leadership.* Boston: Allyn & Bacon.

Scott, A. H. (1999). Wellness works: Community service health promotion groups led by occupational therapy students. *American Journal of Occupational Therapy, 53,* 566-574.

Scott, S. B. (2000, May 22). Community-based fieldwork opportunities: Level I and II experiences. *OT Practice,* 14-18.

Tannenbaum, R. & Schmidt, W. H. (1985). How to choose a leadership pattern. *Harvard Business Review, 36,* 95-101.

Vanier, C. & Hebert, M. (1995). An occupational therapy course on community practice. *Canadian Journal of Occupational Therapy, 62,* 76-81.

Wilson, H. & Kneisel, C. (1988). *Psychosocial nursing concepts and activity book.* Menlo Park, CA: Addison-Wesley.

Yalom, I. (1986). *Theory and practice of group psychotherapy.* New York: Basic Books.

OCCUPATIONAL THERAPY ASSISTANT EDUCATION

The Betty Project:
Jump-Starting Clinical Observation Skills in an OTA Curriculum

Mary Metzger Edwards, RN, OTR

SUMMARY. In the practice environment of many therapy practitioners today, fieldwork educators may have limited time for instructing students in applying basic theoretical concepts. Educators are therefore challenged to develop students who have the tools necessary to be successful in the clinical world.

Based on input from fieldwork educators, the "Betty Project" was developed to provide opportunities for occupational therapy assisting students to hone clinical observation and documentation skills while still in a classroom setting. This modified role-play project gives students an

Mary Metzger Edwards is Instructor and Fieldwork Coordinator, Occupational Therapy Program, University of Southern Indiana, Evansville, IN 47712.

The author gratefully acknowledges the support and assistance of Aimee J. Luebben, EdD, OTR/L, FAOTA, for reading earlier drafts of this article.

[Haworth co-indexing entry note]: "The Betty Project: Jump-Starting Clinical Observation Skills in an OTA Curriculum." Edwards, Mary Metzger. Co-published simultaneously in *Occupational Therapy in Health Care* (The Haworth Press, Inc.) Vol. 15, No. 1/2, 2001, pp. 99-104; and: *Education for Occupational Therapy in Health Care: Strategies for the New Millennium* (eds: Patricia Crist, and Marjorie Scaffa) The Haworth Press, Inc., 2001, pp. 99-104. Single or multiple copies of this article are available for a fee from The Haworth Document Delivery Service [1-800-HAWORTH, 9:00 a.m. - 5:00 p.m. (EST). E-mail address: getinfo@haworthpressinc.com].

opportunity to treat, make clinical observations, and learn to process and prioritize data for effective documentation.

After implementation of this project, student performance in these areas on Level II fieldwork was markedly improved, as evidenced by scores on the FWE as well as fieldwork educator comments. *[Article copies available for a fee from The Haworth Document Delivery Service: 1-800-HAWORTH. E-mail address: <getinfo@haworthpressinc.com> Website: <http://www. HaworthPress.com> © 2001 by The Haworth Press, Inc. All rights reserved.]*

KEYWORDS. Education, clinical observation, documentation

I am Betty. No, you did not misread my byline. For the final 20 weeks of course work each year, I take on an alter ego for the benefit of occupational therapy assisting students to facilitate the strengthening of clinical observation and documentation skills as they work their way towards Level II fieldwork and entry level practice into the field of occupational therapy. This is done in the context of a classroom activity called "The Betty Project."

PURPOSE

The Betty Project was conceived as a tool for providing students with opportunities to put a face on the concepts they have been learning in the occupational therapy assisting curriculum. In the practice environment of many occupational therapy practitioners today, fieldwork educators may not have time for instructing students in applying basic theoretical concepts (Blanchard & Stewart, 2000). Fleming's work (as cited by Neistadt, Wight, & Mulligan, 1998) identifies clinical reasoning as the thought process clinicians use in practice, enabling occupational therapy practitioners to individualize treatment, promote functional performance, and facilitate positive outcomes for their clients. Students, more and more, must be prepared to function and reason in the clinical setting with less of a learning curve than in the past. A "reality gap" often exists between academic expectations and clinical performance (Edwards, 1999). Students engaged in fieldwork may feel self-doubt and concern about their competence (Tryssenaar & Perkins, 2001). Since students primarily engage in the occupations of learning and working within the culture of the classroom early in their education, engaging in these occupations on a variety of levels enables them to achieve a higher degree of organization and confidence. As Yerxa (1998) observed, to engage in occupation is to take control. The Betty Project is designed to funnel concepts of occupation, documentation, clinical observation, clinical reasoning, and related performance components into a practical classroom application. Before they even reach level II fieldwork, occupational therapy assisting students are laying basic groundwork in the functional reality of recognizing and documenting relevant data about clients. The ultimate learning objective of the Betty Project is to advance the skill level of the OTA students in these areas while they are still in the didactic portion of their education, thus "jump-starting" them in preparation for Level II fieldwork.

AN OPPORTUNITY FOR IMPROVEMENT

Feedback from Level II fieldwork educators was the catalyst for the development of the Betty Project. Comments received on the fieldwork evaluation forms identified the need to improve the occupational therapy assistant students' abilities in organizing clinical observations, differentiation between clinically relevant and extraneous information, and students' confidence level in making clinical observations. Another area targeted as needing improvement was that of documenting observations in a thorough and concise manner. Standards for educational programs for occupational therapy assistant students require that students be able to demonstrate the ability to interact via written, oral, and nonverbal communication with colleagues, clients, and others (AOTA, 1999). Focusing on Peloquin and Babola's (1996) discussion of the importance of creating a clinical climate in the classroom, the method to enhance these skills while students were still in the didactic portion of their curriculum became evident.

DESCRIPTION

"The Betty Project," an ongoing role-play beginning the second semester of the first year and continuing through the fourth and final didactic semester of the occupational therapy assistant curriculum, provides a forum for students to hone clinical observation skills and correlate their observations with appropriate documentation. I play the role of Betty, a patient with a diagnosis of cerebral vascular accident, who is followed in our classroom clinic as she progresses from the acute phase of her rehabilitation experience to discharge. Contrary to the initial reaction of several of my colleagues, there is no specific namesake for whom this project is named. *Betty* was chosen because this name crosses a diverse field of age, ethnic, regional, and social contexts. In fact, I have purposefully used this ambiguity to surprise students into examining their own preconceptions: I wait until halfway through the semester when I casually mention Betty's ethnic background, which is different than my own.

This article describes an innovative instructional method where each student, in turn, becomes the treating practitioner during short clinical scenarios while classmates observe and document Betty's response to intervention. Discussion of observed behaviors, as well as ideas for optimal documentation of these clinical observations, occurs afterwards.

IMPLEMENTATION METHOD

At the start of the second semester in the first year of the occupational therapy assisting curriculum, I introduce the students to Betty on paper only. Each student receives a typed summary of the initial occupational therapy evaluation, along with long-term goals and an overview of Betty's occupations, past medical, social, and functional history, and current functional status. I keep this summary very basic, and students are allowed time to review the information in class. I then ask them to identify other information that they think would be necessary or relevant in order to treat Betty. As they start asking questions about Betty, I answer them on the spot–they are clued in that I will be playing the role of Betty–and we add Betty's responses to our database about the client. After we establish all of the relevant data, I inform the students that we will be treating Betty each week in our classroom clinic.

Students are rotated as treating practitioner in alphabetical order for simplicity's sake; they receive their treatment goals several days before the session. Treatment goals each week are based on long-term goals established during the initial evaluation and on Betty's ongoing progress (or lack of progress) towards these goals. The treating student is responsible for developing a treatment idea that addresses the plan. Other students are charged with making clinical observations during the short (five-minute) treatment session. To simplify the process, we focus on sensorimotor treatment ideas incorporated into activities of daily living, work, or leisure areas. Within this scope, students are also reminded to focus on Betty as an occupational being as they plan intervention. Narrowing the focus of treatment is done in the interest of timeliness, since there are restrictions on how much of the class can be devoted to Betty each week.

On the day the student conducts his or her treatment session, Betty's response may vary emotionally or physically. I attempt to make a realistic portrayal of a "typical" patient, while still springing surprises that make the students think on their feet (Peloquin & Babola, 1996). On occasion I may enlist another staff member to play the role of a family member just to keep things interesting.

Following the session, students (including the treating student) take 5-10 minutes to begin writing a progress note including subjective and objective data, as well as their interpretation. After the students complete as much of the progress note as possible in the allotted time, we create a group progress note using transparencies on the overhead projector.

Students keep their progress notes in sequential order in a Betty Notebook. Notebooks are collected and reviewed randomly three times during the semester, noting progress (or lack of progress) in each student's observation and documentation skills. In the Betty Notebook, students keep their original attempt at a note as well as a revision based on the group discussion and progress note. Both versions provide a wealth of information regarding how individual students are processing and prioritizing information, as well as their ability to generalize learning over the course of the project. As the students progress in their abilities, they periodically review each other's notebooks, write constructive criticism, and give positive feedback. Points are assigned for the project based on completion of the Betty Notebook for each treatment session. Students evaluate their overall progress at the end of each semester in the form of a written summary of the process, including identification of improvement made, opportunities for improvement, and ideas for change.

Outcomes

As weeks progress, students generally become more comfortable and proficient at making and documenting clinical observations. Initially, we spend quite a bit of time on basic wording of observations, discussing how to glean and prioritize information, and generally how to process all of the information. Students tend to fixate on minor details, but usually after a few weeks, one student will bring up the revelation that if all this is part of a five- minute session, how much more must be involved in a 30-45 minute session. The most time consuming part of the project is the group progress note. I attempt to limit this phase to 10-15 minutes, but there are times I seize a teachable moment and we use much more time for discussion.

PROJECT OUTCOMES

Prior to implementation of this project, 33% of the students received comments on their Level II fieldwork evaluation indicating that documentation of clinical observations was a deficit area with 0% receiving comments identifying this area as a strength. After the Betty Project was implemented, 47% of the students received comments that identified documentation of clinical observations as an area of strength; no students received comments indicating this was a deficit area. Asked to assess the value of the project at the end of both level II fieldwork experiences, all students (100%) identified the Betty Project as helpful to them and recommended that Betty be kept for future classes.

CONCLUSION

The Betty Project was created and implemented in response to feedback from fieldwork educators indicating that occupational therapy assisting students on Level II fieldwork needed improvement in organizing and documenting clinical observations, as well as prioritizing the clinical relevance of their observations. A comparison of data from fieldwork evaluation forms assessing student performance in these areas before and after the Betty Project was implemented demonstrates that clinical observation skills and documentation skills had shifted from areas of weakness to areas of strength for students on Level II fieldwork. Feedback from students was unanimous in agreeing that the Betty Project was helpful in building their skill levels in these areas.

Providing opportunities for students to hone clinical observation and reasoning skills during the didactic component of the curriculum can increase the confidence, resourcefulness, and flexibility needed to face the challenges of fieldwork and entry-level practice.

REFERENCES

American Occupational Therapy Association (1999). Standards for an accredited educational program for the occupational therapy assistant. *American Journal of Occupational Therapy, 53*, 583-589.

Blanchard, S., & Stewart, C.L. (2000, April 24). Forward chaining: Using standardized patients for clinical education. *OT Practice*, 27-28.

Edwards, M.M. (1999). Stop, drop, and role play: A "think-on-your-feet" classroom strategy. *American Occupational Therapy Association Education Special Interest Section Quarterly, 9*, 3-4.

Neistadt, M.E., Wight, J., & Mulligan, S.E. (1998). Clinical reasoning case studies as teaching tools. *American Journal of Occupational Therapy, 52*, 125-132.

Peloquin, S.M., & Babola, K.A. (1996). Making a clinical climate in the classroom. *American Journal of Occupational Therapy, 50*, 894-898.

Tryssenaar, J., & Perkins, J. (2001). From student to therapist: Exploring the first year of practice. *American Journal of Occupational Therapy, 55*, 19-27.

Yerxa, E.J. (1998). Occupation: The keystone of a curriculum for a self-defined profession. *American Journal of Occupational Therapy, 52*, 365-372.

ACADEMIC LEADERSHIP

A Teacher's Guide
to *The Cheater's Handbook*

Karen Sladyk, PhD, OTR, FAOTA

SUMMARY. Faculty and students come from different eras of scholastic ethics. Students are exposed to vast amounts of information through technology. Enormous pressure to receive high grades leaves students susceptible to the temptations of cheating. Faculty need to be aware of these challenging students and their possible cheating methods so faculty can foster ethical responsibility. *[Article copies available for a fee from The Haworth Document Delivery Service: 1-800-HAWORTH. E-mail address: <getinfo@haworthpressinc.com> Website: <http://www.HaworthPress.com> © 2001 by The Haworth Press, Inc. All rights reserved.]*

KEYWORDS. Cheating, ethics, faculty responsibility

Karen Sladyk is Chair and Professor of Occupational Therapy, Bay Path College, Longmeadow, MA 01106.

[Haworth co-indexing entry note]: "A Teacher's Guide to *The Cheater's Handbook*." Sladyk, Karen. Co-published simultaneously in *Occupational Therapy in Health Care* (The Haworth Press, Inc.) Vol. 15, No. 1/2, 2001, pp. 105-108; and: *Education for Occupational Therapy in Health Care: Strategies for the New Millennium* (eds: Patricia Crist, and Marjorie Scaffa) The Haworth Press, Inc., 2001, pp. 105-108. Single or multiple copies of this article are available for a fee from The Haworth Document Delivery Service [1-800-HAWORTH, 9:00 a.m. - 5:00 p.m. (EST). E-mail address: getinfo@haworthpressinc.com].

Educators experience many highs and a few lows in their academic careers and finding Corbett's (1999) book *The Cheater's Handbook* on display in a national chain bookstore might be considered a low. This small handbook published by Regan Books, a division of HarperCollins, is a how-to book of deception but is labeled for novelty purposes with a tiny 6-point disclaimer on the back cover. Unfortunately, educators will not find this book entertaining.

The book openly states that if students find a topic boring, are stressed, do not test well, do not need the content "in real life," or if the teacher is not engaging, then cheating is an acceptable solution. Despite the obvious ethical issues this book presents, the purpose of this article is to alert faculty to this publication, summarize the recommended cheating techniques, and address practical preventative methods.

One would think that students in Occupational Therapy (OT) or OTA programs would be hesitant to cheat, knowing that all information would "come due" in the NBCOT exam, but, unfortunately, students have reported to me that they have seen NBCOT candidates looking at peers' exams. This might be solved with the new computerized version of the exam, but computers open up other methods for cheating.

In *The Cheater's Handbook,* Corbett (1999) suggests a holistic approach to cheating on papers and exams. Calling in ill or from a "funeral" guarantees everyone else has completed the assigned task. In this approach, additional information is available for the cheater, including possible papers left outside the faculty's office for photocopying and peers sharing test information. Corbett recommends a "uniform" for cheating during exams, including eye glasses to hide eyes, long hair over the face, pullover shirts with a belly pocket to access information by either hand, high topped sneakers, and/or long flowing skirts. The last four items are effective to hide cheat sheets.

Corbett suggests would-be cheaters get copies of lecture notes from another current or former student. Old tests can also be found in a fraternity "scholar's office" or from former students. Even if the teacher changes the tests, the cheater has a style guideline. Corbett cautions students against trying to steal a current exam alone and suggests using work-study students as assistants. He even recommends getting information about a missed exam by using a possible romantic approach with a classmate.

Where and how to sit for exams is fully addressed in chapters six and seven, including figures of typical seating arrangements and positions. Choosing the "right" seat allows for hiding cheat sheets and a backup plan for copying off someone. Cheat sheets should never be more than 4 × 4 inches (2 × 2 recommended) and should be eaten at the first approach of "trouble."

Plagiarism is openly encouraged using old papers, recently corrected papers left outside faculty offices, Internet papers, papers from a chapter, and commercial paper services. *The Cheater's Handbook* lists several commercial paper services that will fax, e-mail, or Fed-ex a completed paper immediately for about $8.00 a page when billed to a credit card. As OT papers are not as readily available commercially, this is less of an issue. However, I have experienced students turning in papers from former and present students without the original author knowing their work has been stolen. In one case, the student turned in last year's old paper taken from a roommate's computer, but included a section that had been removed in the current assignment. In the second case, the original author had tossed her drafts into the recycling bin in the computer center and the cheater simply helped herself. Further investigation found that this was a significant problem, with students routinely removing drafts of assignments from recycling bins.

What can an occupational therapy educator do with so many temptations for cheating? Here are a few suggestions:

- Buy a copy of Corbett's (1999) book, read it, and make it visible in your office.
- Keep all student exams. Allow students access to exams only in your vision. Enter exam scores in your grade book after the exam has been reviewed in class so you know all exams were returned. Another option is to put old exams on reserve in the library for review by everyone.
- Do not leave papers or treatment plans outside your office and encourage other faculty to adopt more secure ways of returning papers. Some students routinely scan faculty hallways for papers or ideas they may use at a later date.
- Mix up the exam room seating and ask students to leave all personal items up against the wall. Scan the room frequently and watch for behaviors outlined in cheating books. Test at the same time as another course test and alternate your students with students taking the other exam.
- Consider two exams for testing day with the same questions but in different order. Copy these on several different color papers and alternate the colors as you pass out the exam.
- Develop a department wide form for late assignment or missed exam permission. Faculty should document each extension request and place the form in the student's file for a comprehensive overview of a potential problem. One teacher, presenting at a local meeting, stated he allows any student to miss any exam for any reason but gives all make-ups on the afternoon of the last day of final exams.
- Advocate for shredders in the computer centers and faculty areas.

- Change the content of treatment plans or papers each year while maintaining the structure so that context becomes the focus.
- Regularly ask students about cheating they may be aware of. Maintain open conversations about ethical issues of importance to students (Reitz, 1997). Address and role model AOTA's Code of Ethics (2000).
- Join your campus academic honesty committee to work at reducing cheating campus-wide.
- Encourage students and faculty to have an open dialogue concerning cheating and the issues raised by both sides.

Students tell me that they appreciate my surveillance and structure around classroom ethics because they feel it keeps a fair and level "playing field" on grading and is positive for our profession.

REFERENCES

American Occupational Therapy Association (2000). *Occupational therapy code of ethics*. Bethesda, MD: Author.

Corbett, B. (1999). *The cheater's handbook*. New York, NY: HarperCollins Publishers.

Reitz, M. (1997). Ethics for students. In K. Sladyk (Ed.), *OT student primer*. Thorofare, NJ: Slack, Inc.

Developing and Maintaining Community Partnerships Within "A Scholarship of Practice"

Brent H. Braveman, MEd, OTR/L
Christine A. Helfrich, PhD, OTR/L
Gail S. Fisher, MPA, OTR/L

SUMMARY. This article describes the application of a model developed and adopted by the occupational therapy faculty at the University of Illinois at Chicago to utilize partnerships with community-based organizations to meet a tripartite mission of education, research, and service delivery. The model (A Scholarship of Practice) was developed and adopted in response to contextual influences occurring at multiple levels. These influences are identified and the actions taken by the faculty are described. "A Scholarship of Practice" is briefly described and the principles that have guided development and maintenance of successful partnerships with community-based organizations are discussed. Finally, the

Brent H. Braveman is Clinical Assistant Professor, Department of Occupational Therapy, University of Illinois at Chicago, 1919 W. Taylor St. (M/C 811), Chicago, IL 60612 (E-mail: Bbravema@uic.edu).

Christine A. Helfrich is Assistant Professor, Department of Occupational Therapy, University of Illinois, Chicago, IL 60612 (E-mail: Helfrich@uic.edu).

Gail S. Fisher is Clinical Assistant Professor, Department of Occupational Therapy, University of Illinois, Chicago, IL 60612 (E-mail: Gfisher@uic.edu).

[Haworth co-indexing entry note]: "Developing and Maintaining Community Partnerships Within 'A Scholarship of Practice.'" Braveman, Brent H., Christine A. Helfrich, and Gail S. Fisher. Co-published simultaneously in *Occupational Therapy in Health Care* (The Haworth Press, Inc.) Vol. 15, No. 1/2, 2001, pp. 109-125; and: *Education for Occupational Therapy in Health Care: Strategies for the New Millennium* (eds: Patricia Crist, and Marjorie Scaffa) The Haworth Press, Inc., 2001, pp. 109-125. Single or multiple copies of this article are available for a fee from The Haworth Document Delivery Service [1-800-HAWORTH, 9:00 a.m. - 5:00 p.m. (EST). E-mail address: getinfo@haworthpressinc.com].

109

outcomes and benefits of partnering with community-based organizations are identified. *[Article copies available for a fee from The Haworth Document Delivery Service: 1-800-HAWORTH. E-mail address: <getinfo@haworthpressinc.com> Website: <http://www.HaworthPress.com> © 2001 by The Haworth Press, Inc. All rights reserved.]*

KEYWORDS. Community-based practice, occupational therapy, curriculum development

INTRODUCTION

The involvement of occupational therapy faculty in community-based organizations is not a new or unique phenomenon (Fazio, 2000; Jackson, Carlson, Mandel, Zemke, & Clark, 1998; Scott, 1999, 2000). However, the decision by an entire occupational therapy faculty to develop longstanding relationships with multiple community-based organizations and to use these relationships as the foundation for curriculum development, research initiatives, and the development and evaluation of clinical service is unique. The occupational therapy faculty at the University of Illinois at Chicago made such a decision. This article will first describe the contextual factors that influenced the faculty to develop and adopt a model of partnering with community-based organizations as part of their efforts to meet their tripartite mission of education, research, and clinical service. Second, the model developed and adopted by the faculty both as a curriculum design, and as a method to guide the involvement of community-based organizations will be presented. Third, the principles used to select and collaborate with community-based organizations are identified and explained. Finally, the outcomes of these collaborations and the benefits for both the faculty and the community-based organizations will be discussed.

A CONTEXT FOR CHANGE

The University of Illinois at Chicago (UIC) is a large urban university with a mission of research, education, and service. A number of contextual factors within the occupational therapy profession and at UIC influenced the faculty in their decision to expand their clinical service mission to partnerships with community-based organizations. These contextual factors combined with the individual interests of the faculty provide a background upon which to frame the model that has since been adopted by the faculty. It is notable that many of these contextual factors were occurring simultaneously rather than sequentially. As a result, the actions taken by the faculty, which are described in the next sections of this article, should be viewed as synergistic responses to the challenges, opportunities, and individual faculty interests.

One influential factor was the increased focus on the development and implementation of community-based practice by occupational therapists (Baum & Law, 1998; Baum & Law, 1997; Braveman, Sen, & Kielhofner, in press; Brownson, 1998; Finlayson & Edwards, 1997; Letts, Fraser, Finlayson, & Walls, 1993; McColl, 1998). While the UIC Department of Occupational Therapy has always been involved in service delivery, the faculty recognized that its scope of involvement in clinical service was primarily limited to hospital-based service, and identified the desire to develop opportunities so that the department's service component would more closely mirror the range of practice occurring in the profession. The faculty also recognized that involvement in community-based settings would facilitate the development of consultative skills and other skill sets that they could then teach more effectively within the curriculum. In addition, they perceived that this involvement could provide opportunities for students for Level I and Level II Fieldwork and for service learning experiences in community-based settings. Service learning is a strategy in which students volunteer in the community or at an organization for academic credit (Scaffa, Van Slyke, & Wooster, 2000).

A second influential factor was the decision by the American Occupational Therapy Association's Representative Assembly in 1999 to require that all occupational therapy educational programs move to post-baccalaureate education by January 2007 (AOTA, 1999). The UIC Occupational Therapy Department had added a Master of Science with Certification program in 1996 to its baccalaureate program. However, the Representative Assembly action required further revision in the curriculum to eliminate baccalaureate education. Only Master of Science students were enrolled in 2000.

Concurrent with these external influences, a synergy began to evolve around research and practice-based collaborations with community-based organizations within the faculty. Two examples of major collaborations included the funding of two research and demonstration projects. One, an Allied Health training grant funded by the Department of Health and Human Services, Health Resources and Services Administration, was a multidisciplinary grant that trained occupational therapy, physical therapy, and human nutrition and dietetic students to work in the community (Helfrich, Fisher, & Kielhofner, 2000). The project was carried out by partnering with six community-based organizations that contributed to the development of the curriculum to train the students and also accepted fieldwork students. The second project, the Employment Options Program, funded by the Department of Education, Rehabilitation Services Administration, developed a vocational rehabilitation program for people with AIDS. This project was conducted in partnership with the Howard Brown Health Center, a community-based health care organization for Chicago's Gay and Lesbian population (Braveman, in press).

A SCHOLARSHIP OF PRACTICE:
A MODEL OF EDUCATION, RESEARCH, AND SERVICE DELIVERY

In response to these multiple influences the faculty began to examine the commonalities in our beliefs around how to respond to the changing environment and redefine our focus. This process included discussions around the nature of scholarship in our department in terms of research, education, and clinical service. It also included discussions of how to integrate the evolving themes of community-based practice and the needs of urban communities into these efforts. The resulting model, "A Scholarship of Practice," has since served to guide us in these endeavors and has become not only a method of describing the commonalities between research efforts, but also guides our curriculum and development of new services.

Through A Scholarship of Practice, we have described scholarship as a dialectic in which theoretical and empirical knowledge is brought to bear on the practical problems of therapeutic work and in which the latter raise questions to be addressed through scholarship. Our scholarship aims to advance the practice of occupational therapy and to make meaningful contributions to interdisciplinary practice. A Scholarship of Practice reflects our university's value of creating knowledge, which addresses and betters the human condition. Our scholarship gives intellectual priority to articulating human problems and critically assessing possible solutions, especially those that relate to the needs of urban communities and urban organizations (Hammel, Finlayson, Kielhofner, Helfrich, & Peterson, submitted manuscript).

Making the decision to partner with other organizations is difficult and complex. Opportunities come from many different avenues, including those initiated by the organization and those initiated by the Occupational Therapy Department. Within each organization are key stakeholders, each of whom may have different interests and goals. Examples of these include organization staff or administration, university faculty or administration, consumers, and students. Deciding which of many potential partnerships to pursue and develop is often a complicated process. Faculty has reflected on how those decisions are made and what we look for in the collaboration. We have articulated principles that guide our thinking about which community-based organizations to include as partners in our scholarship.

PRINCIPLES GUIDING INCLUSION OF COMMUNITY-BASED ORGANIZATIONS IN OUR SCHOLARSHIP EFFORTS

1. Match of Mission Between the Occupational Therapy Department and the Organization

When the department identifies an organization for potential partnership, one of the first issues to analyze is the match between missions. We found that there must be a substantial match for the partnership to develop with shared values and to continue in a mutually beneficial way for both parties. This does not imply that the missions must be identical, but rather that they are complementary and theoretically consistent.

The tripartite mission of the UIC Occupational Therapy Department is broad enough to allow us to find matches with many community-based organizations. Therefore, our task has become one of evaluating the strength and breadth of the match. We look for organizations where the underlying philosophy and the day-to-day service implications of the mission are consistent with ours.

We have learned that the written mission statement often does not adequately reflect the service or operating mission of an organization. Therefore, it is important not to base decisions for potential partnerships on written materials alone. Individual discussions with organization administrators and staff provide an opportunity to understand the organization's mission and to further describe and explain our mission to them. These conversations facilitate understanding of shared values, goals, and needs.

Discussions with representatives of the organization are also an opportunity to educate the organization about occupational therapy. Organizations may have had no prior experience with occupational therapy, or their understanding may be based on previous contact with the field or a practitioner representing either a very specific service or a holistic array of services.

When looking for matches between the department and an organization, it is important to look broadly and creatively within the defined missions. We have found that if we try to stretch the limits of a shared mission too far, the relationship may work initially, but long-term collaborations will be limited.

2. Multifaceted Relationships Work Best

Multifaceted relationships between the organization and the Occupational Therapy Department are the most successful. Multifaceted relationships may include opportunities for education, research, and clinical service. When the relationship encompasses at least two of these components, we have found better matches with our mission and more effective avenues for sustainability. The multifaceted nature of the relationship often provides multiple opportunities for collaboration with multiple staff on both sides.

Multifaceted relationships may provide opportunities for faculty and student research with the organization or its consumers, on-site or classroom educational opportunities, and service opportunities for faculty serving on boards or consulting with staff and students volunteering in the organization. We strive to maximize each relationship without overburdening the organization.

An example of a multifaceted relationship with a domestic violence organization that has developed over eight years involves education, research, and clinical service. One faculty member initially became involved with the organization when asked to write the program evaluation section of a Head Start demonstration project for which they were applying (Beer & Helfrich, 1996). This narrow request led to another faculty member becoming involved in the evaluation that in turn led to a program evaluation with the entire organization. That relationship led to the development of Level I and II fieldwork opportunities, service learning opportunities, service opportunities for faculty serving on the organization's Board of Directors, and ongoing research collaborations for students and faculty between the organization and the Occupational Therapy Department (Walens, Helfrich, Aviles, & Horita, in press).

The strength of the multifaceted relationship is that there are ongoing multiple opportunities for collaboration. If one of those facets is weaker or needs to be terminated, the relationship with the organization does not have to end. Likewise, involvement in more than one aspect of the organization strengthens our ability to educate students with multiple case examples from the same organization, illustrating administration, service, and research in context.

3. Develop a Win-Win Relationship

Limited time and resources make it imperative to invest wisely in relationships that will provide the maximum benefit for both organizations. Venturing into relationships with community-based organizations requires that both the occupational therapy faculty and the community-based organization be willing to define what they hope to achieve by working together. Is the faculty member only looking for a fieldwork site, or is there also an expectation that organization staff will participate in the curriculum via guest lectures and an advisory board? Will there be research collaboration? Is the organization looking for low-cost student help? Do they want programmatic consultation or staff development programs? The faculty member needs to assess mutual needs and desires that could potentially be met by this relationship. Meeting with administrators and staff, conducting focus groups with staff or consumers, and reviewing materials such as the mission statement and annual report are ways to gain information that provides insight into the needs of the organization. Gaining insight into how organizations perceive their effectiveness in meeting their mission, what the organization does very well and not as well, and potential unmet needs provides opportunities to evaluate what occupational therapy has to offer. Through this information gathering, areas of mutual interest are identified where the needs of one of the partners match the skills and resources of the other. The faculty member can describe specific skills and experience relevant to the identified unmet needs and areas for development. Depending on the needs of the organization and the experience of the faculty member, a more extensive needs assessment can be conducted that fully evaluates existing services in the community, consumer and family needs, and the capacity of the organization to develop or modify programs to address unmet needs.

After an initial brainstorming of the possibilities, both the faculty member and organization staff evaluate whether the relationship can be mutually beneficial and is worth pursuing. Initial plans can be summarized in writing, providing the rationale for initiating the relationship, the objectives of it, and the activities that may ensue if the partnership comes to fruition. This type of fact sheet or prospectus provides the organization with something that can be reviewed by the board of directors or staff, insuring that the proposed activities are clearly conveyed. It can also be used to gain support from the Occupational Therapy Department chairperson or the dean, as needed.

4. Evaluate the Feasibility of a Long-Term Partnership

Because we have decided to establish in-depth partnerships with a limited number of community-based organizations, we have found that it is important to evaluate the long-term feasibility of the relationship before going too far with a proposed agreement. Depending on the proposed objectives and activities, the faculty member may want to evaluate the staff's capacity for learning and change, their interest in teaching and providing supervision to students, and their capacity for self-reflection and openness to feedback. Engaging them in telling stories about other collaborative agreements they have had and what did and did not work well may provide some insight in these areas and also may allow the faculty member to assess the organization's openness to outsiders. Reviewing the organization's strategic plan will allow the faculty member to assess whether a long-term relationship is feasible or desirable.

Likewise, the faculty member needs to do a self-assessment about his or her commitment to the organization, and whether the long-term benefits of a partnership warrant a commitment. Is there a good enough fit with the faculty member's values, interests, performance expectations, and career goals to "adopt" the organization and enter into a formal relationship? Faculty may have to provide a lot of up-front effort before seeing the results pay off, and this requires patience and a long-term perspective rather than looking for immediate gains. Providing consultation or student volunteers without asking for anything in return could be considered an investment to show the organization that you are committed to helping them meet their needs, in addition to meeting your own needs.

5. Recognize that Time and Funding Are Venture Capital

Similar to occupational therapy personnel in other settings, academic faculty are feeling increased pressure to meet higher expectations and productivity with fewer resources. In such an environment it can be increasingly difficult to invest time and energy in creative endeavors or new initiatives. A strategy that has promoted success within the UIC Occupational Therapy Department has been the Department Head's decision to allow faculty release time and in some instances to provide financial resources to promote the development of collaborations with community-based organizations. He believes that an investment of initial "venture capital" can in turn have higher payoffs for the department in terms of funded research and educational opportunities (G. W. Kielhofner, personal communication, October, 1997). An example of providing such venture capital led to the eventual submission and funding of the Employment Options Grant previously mentioned. The idea for the program originated at the Howard Brown Health Center. The organization received a small grant to fund development of a program. After a faculty member approached the organization to discuss potential collaborations, the development and evaluation of a pilot program was subcontracted to the UIC Occupational Therapy Department. In turn, the Department Head at UIC set aside two-thirds of the money earned through this subcontract in an account with the understanding that the faculty member could use these funds to aid pursuit of additional grant or foundation funding for the program. In addition, after the initial subcontract was completed, the faculty member was allowed release time to run the program while seeking funding. As a result, a $727,000 federal grant submission was funded, providing considerable salary relief for the department. Similar practices have resulted in the development of partnerships with other organizations.

Another successful model has been to obtain external or internal grant funds to cover part of faculty time for starting community partnerships. This investment of funds is often enough to provide release from some existing duties and to allow more time to identify and work with potential community-based organization collaborators. Once those relationships are in place, the funding can be replaced by new sources or the cost for maintaining the relationship can be absorbed by either the organization or the university, since the payoffs are evident by that point.

6. Maintain a Single Point of Contact to Facilitate Communication

Establishing and maintaining trust is critical to the long-term survival of any partnership. The faculty has found this to be especially true in their collaborations with community-based organizations. A key time in the process of establishing trust within a relationship is during the early stages when confusion and miscommunication may cause irreparable damage. To avoid this we adopted the principle that there should be one faculty member who initially serves as a single point of contact with each community-based organization. The purpose of having a single point of contact is not to exclude involvement of other faculty at an organization, but to ensure that staff and key decision-makers at the organization know whom to contact if there are questions or problems. Early in the relationship, many questions arise about roles and responsibilities and there may be the need for troubleshooting in a timely and effective manner if problems or misunderstandings arise. Examples of issues that have needed attention have been questions about contracts or insurance when service provision is involved, overcoming resistance of staff who are not sure why faculty members or students are at the organization, and clarifying what is or is not appropriate for occupational therapists to address. As relationships develop and change over time, it has also been helpful for a single faculty member to accept responsibility for renegotiating agreements or responsibilities. Finally, maintaining a single point of contact has allowed us to use faculty time in an efficient manner and develop significant partnerships with multiple organizations while maintaining healthy relationships with each.

7. Establish Clear Expectations Regarding the Nature of the Relationship

It is important to build an effective working relationship by clearly defining roles, responsibilities, and expectations, and by specifying and measuring outcomes. Once the faculty member identifies the key staff to work with, relationship building can occur. Activities to facilitate this include spending time at the organization observing the culture, norms, and environment of the organization, formally or informally interviewing staff members (if not already completed during the initial phase), shadowing staff to get a better idea of what they do, and finding out what is most important to the staff and the consumers of the organization's services. In-depth discussion to gain insight into each other's worlds will help to build the relationship. This can include sharing relevant priorities, values, frustrations, success stories, resources and rewards. Mutual respect develops over time and with ongoing dialogue about common concerns. In this initial phase, there should be discussions about the frequency and mode of communication. Ongoing communication occurring on a regular basis is key to both establishing and maintaining the relationship.

Initially, it is expected that some rough spots will lead to redefining the relationship. However, difficulties can be minimized by clearly defining expectations up front. Commitments of time, resources and expertise should be clear and mutually agreed upon. Each partner should feel comfortable saying, "I can't do that." For each type of collaboration, such as student training or research participation, roles and responsibilities of both the faculty member and the organization staff should be spelled out. We have developed guidelines for the roles of faculty, agency staff, and students (Walens et al., in press).

Both the faculty member and the organization staff should define expected outcomes. Mutually agreed-upon outcomes should be put into writing, along with timelines, persons responsible, and criteria for evaluation, and should be shared with all involved parties. These outcomes may be products, such as a program manual or a revised staff training module; they may be accomplishments, such as a certain number of students completing fieldwork or a certain number of staff or consumers who provide guest lectures for the curriculum; they may be supportive of each other's goals, such as letters of support provided for grant submissions or becoming an advisory board member; or they may be joint publications or presentations at professional meetings or community consortia. There may also be some process outcomes, such as staff feeling increased comfort with the faculty member, students being accepted by the organization, or an increased perception that the relationship feels truly collaborative and mutually beneficial.

8. Maintain the Relationship Over Time

Maintaining the relationship between the Occupational Therapy Department and the organization includes ongoing reevaluation of benefits, renegotiation of roles, flexibility, and capitalizing on unanticipated opportunities. Because we strive to develop long-term relationships with organizations, we assume from the start that we will need to reevaluate and renegotiate those relationships. This requires thoughtfully considering the long-term benefits of the partnership which sometimes involves placing emphasis on the organization's needs instead of our own.

When faculty, students, and the organization's staff identify problems, concerns, or potential opportunities, they must be discussed. Issues may arise due to changes in the organization's mission or direction, consumer needs, the occupational therapy curriculum, faculty resources, or student needs. Any of these changes may affect both parties positively or negatively resulting in further development or termination of a partnership.

It is often difficult to terminate, or place on hold, a partnership with an organization if the relationship has been positive. The department must assess the ongoing benefits and the available resources in making such decisions. For example, the decision to place a partnership on hold may occur even if the organization has been considered beneficial for student training if there are not available faculty resources to supervise students and maintain the relationship. The same decision could be made on the part of the organization if the resources needed or the priorities of the organization significantly outweighed the benefit of having university involvement. In either case, the department recognizes its dynamic and evolving research and service nature and may renegotiate a new relationship in the future if it will be mutually beneficial.

The process of relationship maintenance may involve the renegotiation of roles. Faculty may increase or broaden their involvement with an organization and organizational staff may do the same with the Occupational Therapy Department. As noted in earlier examples, relationships commonly start off in one or two areas and then broaden to become multifaceted over time to meet multiple needs. Faculty may expand their involvement to assume multiple roles such as researcher, student supervisor, and board member, or additional individuals may come on board to assume expanding roles. Likewise organization staff may take on the additional roles of data collectors, student supervisors, guest lecturers, or grant collaborators. At each stage of role renegotiation discussion needs to be honest and open to understand the implications and concerns of all involved. This allows proactive problem solving and any needed resource allocation. The worst possible outcome is for a faculty or staff member to agree to something that is not valued or feasible out of a sense of obligation.

Another issue to consider is remaining alert for unexpected benefits that may arise for either partner. Sometimes opportunities for collaboration may occur that were unanticipated through discussion between partners or through discussions one partner may have with third parties about his or her own work within the organization. The lesson we have learned is that it is often worth exploring the feasibility of the ideas before making a decision. An example of an unanticipated benefit occurred when the American Occupational Therapy Association approached a faculty member working with a domestic violence organization about evaluating a demonstration project for school violence prevention with children and families (M. Scheinholtz, personal communication, April 3, 2000). She approached the domestic violence organization to see if they were interested in participating. To her surprise, the collaboration expanded to allow families served by the organization to participate in the program, staff to receive training as program leaders, graduate students to develop thesis proposals to expand the program evaluation, and students to obtain education and deliver community service as program assistants!

The process of maintaining the relationship may seem overly simple at times, and absolutely untenable at others. Both partners need to consider the long-term outcomes when determining how much time, energy, and resources should be placed on relationship maintenance. While the benefits of this work can be incredible, in some cases the difficult decision to end the relationship may also need to be made.

OUTCOMES AND BENEFITS

We have found that the outcomes and benefits of including community-based organizations as an integral part of our Scholarship of Practice have been well worth the investment of resources in terms of time and funding. The following section of this article provides a brief description of the varied outcomes and benefits realized by the faculty.

1. Fieldwork and Service Learning Opportunities

Students have been placed with our community-based organization partners for fieldwork. Faculty have been involved in the supervision in different ways. One faculty member volunteered to supervise Level I students at a shelter for families fleeing domestic violence as a strategy to further develop a relationship. Later, this supervision was paid for by the UIC Occupational Therapy Department. A second faculty member has negotiated with a supportive living residence for people with AIDS to supervise Level II students by going on-site one day a week. Part of this experience included the faculty member and the students collaborating on program development for the organization. In return, the organization reimbursed the UIC Occupational Therapy Department for the faculty member's time. Post-professional master's students have also provided on-site supervision for entry-level MS students as a teaching practicum or part of a graduate assistantship. Recently, we expanded our ongoing presence in the organizations by placing small groups of students for a three-hour per week service learning experience at each of the six organizations with whom we are currently partnering. At UIC, the focus of the student's experiences changes each semester to match the emphasis of classroom learning that semester.

2. Master's Projects and Thesis Topics

At UIC we utilize a model of student scholarship in which students are assigned topics for their final projects or theses by their advisors. We have found that this approach provides students with structured support and focus, while making a contribution to a broader tradition of scholarship by building on prior work (Hammel, Finlayson, Kielhofner, Helfrich, & Peterson, in press). Some project or thesis topics are chosen in collaboration with organization personnel or with the previously identified needs of our organization partners in mind. This has been viewed as a payoff for the time and resources that the organization contributes to the supervision of students during their service learning or fieldwork experiences at the organizations. An example of a Master's project would include the development of a workbook to help people with AIDS, who are transitioning from supported to independent living situations, to learn to grocery shop while on a budget. Other examples include developing an intake or follow-up screening tool to be used by organization staff and consumers. An example of a Master's thesis would include analysis of data collected as part of a needs assessment of homeless women fleeing domestic violence, to make recommendations for program development.

3. Assignments Tied to Specific Courses

As faculty attempt to involve the students in active learning, they often create assignments requiring students to interact with consumers of occupational therapy. Community-based organizations can be used as learning laboratories for assignments that require application of classroom learning. For example, one course at UIC included an assignment for students to provide Internet training for older adults at a local senior center. Another course required students to work with community-living adults with disabilities who were trying to improve their living or work situation. The students worked in small teams with a consumer from one of our organization partners, and they performed several person and environment assessments that they had learned in that course. They helped the consumer to develop a community-living goal and then assisted them with locating community resources to address that goal.

4. Funded Research and Support for Grants

We have partnered with community-based organizations in a number of ways related to funded research and submission of grant applications. Our community-based organization partners have assisted us with submission of grant applications by writing letters of support, allowing us to collect pilot data, and helping to make connections with other organizations in the community that strengthen the quality of the proposal. Once funded, we have partnered with community-based organizations to carry out both research and demonstration endeavors. We have experienced considerable success with this strategy, obtaining over $1.5 million dollars in federal research and demonstration funding over a four-year period.

5. Curriculum Development

In addition to becoming a major focus of our new curriculum design, our community-based partners have assisted with curriculum development and improvement in a number of ways. Organization personnel have collaborated with faculty to identify suggestions for content for both our core curriculum and elective courses offered in the department. Many of the same personnel and some consumers of organization services have participated in the curriculum as guest speakers. Recent graduates also share their experiences in the community-based organizations with students preparing to enter those settings.

6. Faculty Development

Because faculty involvement in community-based organizations has been quite varied, the faculty has had the opportunity to both keep skills current and to develop new skills. The community partnerships provide faculty with an opportunity to operationalize their interests in a manner that supports their scholarship and teaching. In fact, potential faculty members who apply for positions are now informed that there is an expectation that each faculty member will work with at least one community-based organization of their choosing for education, research, or service purposes. This is evidence of the culture that supports these partnerships and how they are seen as integral to faculty success.

Faculty experiences at the organizations can be utilized as case examples that represent service in evolving settings and reflect the current challenges experienced by clinicians and organizations alike. An example of this integration includes the development of a series of three courses in the curriculum that are titled "Synthesis I, II and III." These courses utilize a problem-based learning approach relying on cases, many of which are pulled from recent faculty experience at community-based organizations. Faculty have also been able to improve or develop new skill sets such as consultative and program development skills that directly relate to content required by accreditation standards for occupational therapy programs (AOTA, 2000).

7. Service Delivery Missions of Both Organizations

The UIC Occupational Therapy Department partnerships with community-based organizations have assisted us with our service delivery mission in a number of ways. First, service has been provided in the context of fieldwork. Second, some faculty have provided service within organizations on a contractual basis. Because faculty are somewhat autonomous in managing their schedules and because service delivery is not their primary mission, they have been able to negotiate contracts with our partners to provide limited services on an as-needed basis. This type of arrangement benefits organizations that may not have sufficient need or resources to hire a permanent, full-time occupational therapist. We only ask to be reimbursed for our expenses without concern about financial profit; although salary recovery has helped with measures of productivity for faculty, and the department always finds use for the extra funds.

8. Benefits and Outcomes for the Community-Based Organization

We previously identified that establishing a "win-win" situation for both the UIC Occupational Therapy Department and our community-based partners is one principle that has guided our actions. The benefits of our relationship are as varied for our community-based partners as they are for us and are both tangible and symbolic in nature. Some of the tangible benefits include the program enhancements, student projects, and client services already mentioned. In addition, when grants or other funded research are conducted at a community-based organization, a portion of the salary for one or more organization personnel is usually reimbursed for the period of the grant. We have reimbursed organizations by writing staff into projects, as co-investigators or other paid positions. Two of our organization partners have also benefited by hiring graduates of the occupational therapy program who became aware of the organization as students because of our partnership. The benefits which are more symbolic in nature, but nonetheless important, included the perceived status, for both the organization and individual organization personnel, of affiliation with a university and university sponsored education and research activities, and the opportunity to contribute to preparation of students for the future in evolving service areas.

CONCLUSION

We have noted in this article that our decision to develop and maintain partnerships with community-based organizations to aid us in our missions of education, research, and service delivery has required considerable effort and commitment. In order to be successful, faculty have had to be willing to commit to extra effort, both at the initiation of a new partnership and as the partnership grows and changes, in order to maintain the relationship over time. It must be reemphasized, however, that the benefits gained have been numerous, varied, and have proven to be well worth the effort. We also recognize that we will face additional challenges in the future.

We anticipate that continuation of this model will require ongoing attention to funding issues by both the Occupational Therapy Department and our community-based partners. Universities, faculty, and community-based organizations are challenged by increased competition for limited resources, and future success will depend upon our abilities to meet these challenges by remaining energized, flexible, and creative.

Finally, we recognize that that we will need to participate in continuous curriculum evaluation to measure the impact of our partnerships and the experiences they provide for students on program outcomes. As we introduced this article we spoke of a "context for change" and the many forces that influenced our decision to embark on the process of partnering with community-based organizations. We expect that we will continue to be influenced by factors in the environments of our profession, our university, and the communities in which our partners are located. Continued success will demand diligence and creativity to effectively respond to the yet unknown influences we will face in the future.

AUTHOR NOTE

The authors would like to acknowledge the other members of the UIC faculty who were integral to the efforts described in this article, including Gary Kielhofner, Joy Hammel, Debra Walens, Elizabeth Peterson, and Marcia Finlayson. We would also like to acknowledge and thank the staff and consumers at all of our community-based organization partners who have worked so hard to make these partnerships a success. We also must acknowledge the Department of Education, Rehabilitation Services Administration for their funding of project H235A980170, the Department of Health and Human Services, Health Resources and Services Administration for their funding of project 5D37AH00607, and the Department of Education, National Institute on Disability and Rehabilitation Research for their funding of Project H133G990144.

REFERENCES

American Occupational Therapy Association (2000). Standards for an accredited educational program for the occupational therapist. In *The Reference Manual of the Official Documents of the American Occupational Therapy Association, Inc., Eighth Edition.* Bethesda, MD: American Occupational Therapy Association.

American Occupational Therapy Association (1999). ACOTE sets timeline for post-baccalaureate degree programs. *OT Week, 13,* 33.

Baum, C., & Law, M. (1998). Nationally speaking-community health: A responsibility, an opportunity, and a fit for occupational therapy. *The American Journal of Occupational Therapy, 52* (1), 7-10.

Baum, C., & Law, M. (1997). Occupational therapy practice: Focusing on occupational performance. *The American Journal of Occupational Therapy, 51,* 277-288.

Beer, D., & Helfrich, C. (1996). Evaluation of Ridgeland Enhanced Head Start Program for Transitional Housing Residents. Final Report, U.S. Department of Health and Human Services.

Braveman, B.H. (in press). Development of a community-based return to work program for people with AIDS. *Occupational Therapy in Health Care.*

Braveman, B.H., Sen, S., & Kielhofner, G. (in press). Community-based vocational rehabilitation programs. In M. Scaffa (Ed.) *Occupational Therapy in Community-Based Practice Settings.* Philadelphia: F.A. Davis.

Brownson, C.A. (1998). Funding community practice: Stage 1. *The American Journal of Occupational Therapy, 52* (1), 60-64.

Fazio, L. (2000). *Developing Occupation-Centered Programs for the Community: A Workbook for Students and Professionals.* Upper Saddle River, NJ: Prentice-Hall.

Finlayson, M., & Edwards, J. (1997). Evolving health environments and occupational therapy: Definitions, descriptions and opportunities. *The British Journal of Occupational Therapy, 60* (10), 456-459.

Hammel, J., Finlayson, M., Kielhofner, G., Helfrich, C., & Peterson, E.W. Educating scholars of practice: An approach to preparing tomorrow's researchers. Manuscript submitted for publication.

Helfrich, C., Fisher, & Kielhofner, G. (2000). Definitions of allied health services in urban community contexts: Consumer perspectives. *Journal of Allied Health, 29,* 71-78.

Jackson, J., Carlson, M., Mandel, D., Zemke, R., & Clark, F. (1998). Occupation in lifestyle redesign: The well elderly study occupational therapy program. *The American Journal of Occupational Therapy, 52,* 326-336.

Letts, L., Fraser, B., Finlayson, M., & Walls, J. (1993). *For the Health of It! Occupational Therapy Within a Health Promotion Framework.* Toronto: CAOT Publications ACE.

McColl, M.A. (1998). What do we need to know to practice occupational therapy in the community. *The American Journal of Occupational Therapy, 52* (1), 11-18.

Scaffa, M., Van Slyke, N., & Wooster, D.M. (2000). A community service learning approach to Level I fieldwork: An investment in the future. In P. Christ (Ed.) *Innovations in Occupational Therapy Education.* Bethesda, MD: The American Occupational Therapy Association, Inc.

Scott, A.H. (1999). Wellness works: Community service health promotion groups led by occupational therapy students. *The American Journal of Occupational Therapy, 53,* 566-574.

Scott, S. (2000). Community-based fieldwork opportunities: Level I and II experiences. *OT Practice,* May 22, 2000, 14-18.

Walens, D., Helfrich, C.A., Aviles, A., & Horita, L. (in press). Assessing needs and developing interventions with new populations: A community process of collaboration. *Occupational Therapy in Mental Health.*

Combining Roles as an Academic Instructor and a Clinical Practitioner in Occupational Therapy: Benefits, Challenges, and Strategies for Success

Albert E. Copolillo, PhD, OTR/L
Elizabeth Walker Peterson, MPH, OTR/L
Christine A. Helfrich, PhD, OTR/L

SUMMARY. Approximately 28% of the total occupational therapy (OT) faculty in higher education are adjunct faculty members. Adjunct faculty (i.e., faculty who teach a course or part of a course) have been used in higher education to maintain quality educational experiences while providing positive community connections and educational resources with first-hand experience. In occupational therapy, practitioners often assume adjunct faculty responsibilities, thereby significantly increasing professional workloads. Despite added effort, there are sev-

Albert E. Copolillo is Assistant Professor, Department of Occupational Therapy at Virginia Commonwealth University. Address correspondence to: P.O. Box 980008, Richmond, VA 23298-0008.

Elizabeth Walker Peterson is Clinical Assistant Professor and Christine A. Helfrich is Assistant Professor, both from the Department of Occupational Therapy at the University of Illinois at Chicago, 1919 West Taylor Street (M/C 811), Chicago, IL 60612.

[Haworth co-indexing entry note]: "Combining Roles as an Academic Instructor and a Clinical Practitioner in Occupational Therapy: Benefits, Challenges, and Strategies for Success." Copolillo, Albert E., Elizabeth Walker Peterson, and Christine A. Helfrich. Co-published simultaneously in *Occupational Therapy in Health Care* (The Haworth Press, Inc.) Vol. 15, No. 1/2, 2001, pp. 127-143; and: *Education for Occupational Therapy in Health Care: Strategies for the New Millennium* (eds: Patricia Crist, and Marjorie Scaffa) The Haworth Press, Inc., 2001, pp. 127-143. Single or multiple copies of this article are available for a fee from The Haworth Document Delivery Service [1-800-HAWORTH, 9:00 a.m. - 5:00 p.m. (EST). E-mail address: getinfo@haworthpressinc.com].

eral benefits to adjunct teaching. However, there are equally as many challenges.

Objectives of this article were to describe rewards and challenges of adjunct teaching and suggest strategies for successfully negotiating adjunct roles. The article summarizes findings from needs assessments undertaken to develop adjunct faculty programs. Results are relevant to practitioners with both clinical and teaching roles, and to their supervisors and peers. *[Article copies available for a fee from The Haworth Document Delivery Service: 1-800-HAWORTH. E-mail address: <getinfo@ haworthpressinc.com> Website: <http://www.HaworthPress.com> © 2001 by The Haworth Press, Inc. All rights reserved.]*

KEYWORDS. Adjunct professors, faculty, part-time faculty

In 1997, 411 adjunct faculty members were employed in occupational therapy (OT) programs, comprising 28% of the total occupational therapy faculty (i.e., both COTA and OTR programs) (AOTA, 1997). Although the number of occupational therapy (OT) programs granted developing program status is slowing, the rapid development of new programs in the 1990s has resulted in an urgent need for qualified instructors. Currently, the American Occupational Therapy Association's Accreditation Council accredits 136 occupational therapy programs and 178 occupational therapy assistant programs for OT education (ACOTE).

Adjunct faculty, defined as instructors who teach a course or part of a course in a higher education program, have made valuable contributions to academic OT programs and will likely remain an integral part of most departments. In addition to providing clinical expertise, employing adjunct faculty members may help to free tenured and tenure-track faculty to engage in research that will expand the profession's knowledge base. In 1978, the Ad Hoc Committee on Education of the American Occupational Therapy Association recommended that OT faculty redistribute energies by reducing, delegating, and handling activities more efficiently to increase their time commitment to research and scholarly work (Johnson, 1978).

Results of a study by Parham (1987) indicate that only 19% of faculty feel they have sufficient time to conduct research. The low publication rates of OT faculty relative to overall rates in higher education place OT faculty in a vulnerable position (Parham, 1985). Thus, there continues to be a need to help academic departments manage the challenge of facilitating clinical excellence among entry-level students and scholarly excellence among faculty hired to conduct research. Exploring the nature of adjunct faculty positions and assisting OT practitioners to develop strategies for success in these roles is beneficial for both individuals and the profession.

The purpose of this article is to discuss the benefits and challenges of adjunct faculty positions in OT programs. Its goal is to foster success in adjunct faculty positions by offering practitioners strategies for proactively addressing the challenges associated with those positions.

LITERATURE REVIEW

Within academic settings and across disciplines, the use of adjunct faculty has been debated. Colleges and universities employ adjunct faculty as a way to improve or augment high quality education. These institutions often accomplish advanced educational goals through use of adjunct faculty while reducing costs and increasing control over human resources (Gappa & Leslie, 1993; Leatherman, 1997; Tuckman, 1978). Many institutions take pride in incorporating professionals working in the community into their programs. However, colleges and universities with disproportionately high numbers of adjunct and part-time faculty relative to the number of full-time faculty, throughout the institution or within a single academic unit, have sometimes been criticized for the quality of their programs. An often identified disadvantage to employing adjuncts is their limited availability for non-teaching duties, i.e., advising, curriculum planning, and committee work (Rhoades, 1996; Tuckman, 1978).

Professionals from a variety of academic disciplines report seeking adjunct faculty positions for many reasons. Studies indicate that many are attracted by a flexible, part-time schedule that provides an opportunity to remain active in their fields while maintaining other primary role responsibilities (Gappa & Leslie, 1993). Some individuals see adjunct positions as stepping-stones to full-time academic positions, as a way of varying work responsibilities, or as a means of providing added financial support. At the same time, these same instructors have identified a lack of job security, marginal status, and a limited sense of involvement and participation in curriculum planning as barriers to job satisfaction (Gappa & Leslie, 1993; Tuckman, 1978). The underlying reasons for choosing an adjunct faculty position can often explain one's ultimate job satisfaction and success. For example, if one chooses an adjunct role over a more desirable full-time faculty position to avoid relocating, there may be an increased risk of feeling dissatisfied in the adjunct role. Despite these concerns, many adjunct faculty members report finding their positions rewarding.

To the authors' knowledge, there are no discussions of the special needs of adjunct faculty in OT programs who also work as practitioners. However,

Brayley (1996) makes several general suggestions for OT practitioners considering a switch to an academic career, which, while not specifically directed toward adjunct faculty, may be helpful to those in adjunct roles.

This article was written to identify the many benefits and challenges of being an adjunct faculty member. The subject is relevant not only to the OT practitioners who are combining teaching and clinical roles but also to the individuals who supervise and work with them. This article summarizes findings from needs assessments undertaken by two occupational therapy educational programs in Research 1 universities. The needs assessments were conducted to develop adjunct faculty development programs. Through this article, the authors suggest ways of increasing the likelihood for success in combined teaching and practicing roles.

In order to gain a greater understanding of the roles of adjunct faculty members and as part of an administrative examination of faculty needs, the authors interviewed seven occupational therapy practitioners who have assisted with teaching or have been responsible for full courses in OT academic programs. The authors used a 48-item structured interview that was adapted from a questionnaire designed by Gappa and Leslie (1993). This structured interview was designed to describe the experience of an adjunct faculty member. The authors sought to understand the amount of time spent preparing to teach; reasons for teaching; career aspirations; type of orientation and mentoring provided; and level of satisfaction with adjunct teaching. These therapists were also asked to list the greatest benefits and drawbacks to adjunct faculty positions. The questionnaire consisted of a combination of structured response choice and open-ended questions. Two additional sources were used to develop this article: (1) literature discussing trends in higher education and describing the roles and functions of adjunct faculty across disciplines, and (2) group interviews with occupational therapy educators and practitioners.

BENEFITS TO COMBINING TEACHING AND PRACTICE IN OT

Flexible Hours

One of the advantages to working in adjunct positions is the opportunity to work part-time. Many adjunct faculty have a combination of both part-time clinical and teaching positions, which serve to create greater diversity of job activities and responsibilities. Part-time status allows for opportunities to acquire income while freeing time for other valued activities, including responsibilities at home and in the community. Part-time work is often attractive to semi-retired individuals because it provides the opportunity to continue to practice without having to spend 35 or more hours at a workplace. Some therapists find being able to prepare courses at home complementary to their lifestyles and schedules.

Income

Income is seldom the sole reason for becoming an adjunct faculty member, but it is an important consideration. Income generated from part-time teaching activities can serve to supplement that generated from clinical practice. In some cases, practitioners may teach in academic programs affiliated with their primary employer (e.g., a medical center). In these situations, practitioners may not receive direct payment for their teaching. Instead, clinical departments might be paid by the academic department in order to allow release time, i.e., time away from the clinical setting for a practitioner to contribute to the educational program.

Assessing Academia

Adjunct teaching provides an entry-point to the academic world. It gives practitioners an opportunity to evaluate whether an academic career is desirable. Occupational therapy and OT assistant programs typically use diverse educational methods (e.g., lectures, Websites, labs). Therefore, practitioners have multiple venues to explore teaching. For example, many academic program directors are eager to provide local practitioners with the opportunity to assist with the lab section of a course or to teach a single module within a larger course. This allows the OT practitioner an opportunity to experience a variety of teaching situations before making any longer-term commitments to more complex adjunct teaching responsibilities.

Working as an adjunct faculty member provides the OT practitioner with access to university or community college resources, such as libraries and computer technology laboratories. Working as an adjunct is also a good way to develop collaborative alliances or mentoring relationships with full-time academicians in OT. This can be a valuable way for a practitioner who is considering pursuing an advanced degree to get to know faculty and explore the academic environment while building skills that may be helpful during and after graduate school. Experiences as an adjunct faculty member in an accredited school can often be applied toward the fulfillment of teaching requirements associated with advanced degree programs.

Facilitating Professional Growth

Developing and teaching a course requires several of the leadership, organization, and planning skills necessary for advancement in the profession. Additionally, if a practitioner already possesses these skills, accepting an adjunct faculty position may be a valuable opportunity to put them to use. Once an individual is recognized as a resource for a particular topic or set of topics, other practice and academic opportunities may become available because teaching skills can be applied to a variety of settings. Success in teaching may build confidence and willingness to try other new professional ventures.

Informing and Invigorating Practice

Adjunct teaching responsibilities include reading and reviewing literature and following new developments in the field. Instructors are required to organize materials and create a framework for covering the material. Classroom discussions may give rise to new insights on practice, and contact with other faculty may lead to discovering new sources of data and information. An academic teaching experience may put a new perspective on other professional interests. For example, teaching may make a practitioner more aware of the link between theory and practice, thereby fostering a more reflective practice that creates new professional interests. As an adjunct faculty member gets feedback and questions from students, he/she may be forced to examine the efficacy of intervention approaches and techniques. This may lead to rethinking practice habits and decision-making processes. Therefore, an OT practitioner can use adjunct faculty experiences to analyze her/his practice and make changes that reflect a more in-depth understanding of occupational therapy concepts.

Personal Satisfaction

Many practitioners describe a sense of personal satisfaction from adjunct teaching. They feel that the time spent with students in classrooms or labs is dynamic and the energy derived from such an enlivening experience transfers to other roles and responsibilities. Satisfaction comes from making a contribution to an educational program and to the profession at large. Occupational therapy practitioners strengthen academic programs by bringing current clinical expertise and reasoning skills into the classroom. In addition to informing students of practice trends, practitioners can draw from their day-to-day experiences to discuss the impact of changes in service delivery systems and reimbursement on practice. In other words, practitioners have access to real cases and can create educational activities that offer a practical and context-specific perspective. Positive feedback received from students can increase a practitioner's confidence and appreciation for her/his role as a practitioner.

CHALLENGES TO ADJUNCT FACULTY IN OCCUPATIONAL THERAPY

Limited Status and Job Security

By their nature, adjunct faculty positions lack security and can be lower status positions within an academic program. This may be the major disadvantage to working as an adjunct faculty member. The adjunct faculty position offers flexibility not only for the employee but also for the program director, who typically maintains extensive managerial discretion over any part-time position. A major source of this discretion is often the omission of conditions regarding appointment and release. In addition, wages may not always be influenced by teaching experience, so adjunct faculty who maintain teaching positions for extended periods cannot necessarily expect regular increases in their wages (Gappa & Leslie, 1993).

Orientation to the OT Department

Often, new adjunct faculty do not know what they need to know to perform their responsibilities efficiently. In some situations, the need for a more thorough orientation only becomes apparent after the adjunct faculty member makes an unusual request, fails to follow a standard operating procedure, or is unable to get her/his needs met. Although thorough orientations can relieve the stress associated with adjunct teaching, they are not always provided in academic programs.

The Labor Intensive Nature of the First Year

First-time teaching is time-consuming and labor intensive. Preparing to teach a course for the first time can be at least twice as time-consuming as repeating the same course a second time because preparation involves mastering the topics to be presented, outlining and scheduling lectures and labs, and preparing and copying handouts and exams. New educators must learn a variety of new skills simultaneously, making the first time one teaches a course especially challenging. Therefore, the initial investment in course preparation pays off when one has the opportunity to repeat the course. Since adjunct faculty are not guaranteed continuous teaching responsibilities, they are at risk for not getting a return on their invested time and effort.

Formal Evaluation and Informal Feedback

Involvement in well-developed systems for evaluation of performance should be one of the highest priorities for adjunct faculty. However, receiving timely, constructive feedback from students and supervisors is a challenge to adjunct faculty members for at least two reasons. First, because program directors often have discretion over whether and how to evaluate adjunct faculty, feedback on performance may be delayed or nonexistent. Second, adjunct faculty spend less time in a department than full-time faculty. If students have limited opportunities to meet with the adjunct faculty member outside of class, they may be unable to express concerns about the structure or content of the course until completing course evaluations at the end of the semester. When feedback comes at the end of a course, the adjunct faculty member has fewer, if any, opportunities to remedy problems and get clarification on the feedback. Adjunct faculty members who have not mastered the management of teacher-student relationships and receive overwhelmingly negative feedback from students or supervisors are likely to perceive teaching as unrewarding. Untimely feedback and course evaluations reduce adjunct faculty members' opportunities to engage in conflict resolution when necessary, and thereby build teaching skills.

Unless criteria for evaluation of overall performance are identified, it can be challenging for the adjunct faculty member to learn the expectations and values in the academic system. Academic managers may regard certain expectations as inherent in the role of any instructor in the department, but the adjunct faculty member may not recognize them as part of her/his responsibilities. In the needs assessments conducted by the authors, expectations that were not clearly articulated by academic directors included involvement with curriculum and program evaluation, student remediation, student advising, effective use of new audiovisual technologies, communication via e-mail, and involvement in online chats with students.

Limited Peer Contact

Because they must move between at least two settings, adjunct faculty who are also practitioners may have little time to make contact with other faculty in the OT program. Adjunct faculty members may not always have enough time to check in with other instructors to find out how students are applying the material they are teaching. If adjunct faculty members are unable to attend faculty meetings, they may have little opportunity to influence decisions that might have an impact on their course(s) and job status.

Contact with clinical practice peers can also be limited by the need to move between clinical and academic settings. For example, teacher-practitioners may find they have less time to process concerns about challenging patients with their peers, or they may be unable to participate in important patient referral or scheduling decisions with the rest of the staff.

Meeting the Needs and Expectations of More than One Employment Setting

Being accountable to more than one employer may require the teacher-practitioner to overcompensate in demonstrating competency and accountability in both academic and practice settings. Practitioners who negotiate with their clinical supervisors to change from full-time to part-time status or to get release time to teach may be especially vulnerable. In most clinical environments, practicing and teaching is not the norm, so the clinical performance of the teacher-practitioner may be more closely scrutinized than that of her/his peers. If a new adjunct faculty member is unaware of the extensive amount of preparation time needed to teach a new course, he/she may have difficulty managing time effectively. Consequently, the new adjunct may have to resort to using personal time to complete job responsibilities. Prolonged sacrificing of free time is likely to have a negative impact on job performance and may eventually lead to burnout. Adjunct faculty may also experience resentment from peers whose job responsibilities were increased to accommodate release time or schedule changes for the adjunct.

Minor Annoyances

Several of the adjunct faculty members the authors talked with referred to concerns with their roles as "minor annoyances" or "little things." These minor annoyances: inadequate office space and computer access; not being informed or being notified later than full-time faculty of class cancellations; not receiving paychecks on time; not having a place to secure personal belongings (e.g., a locker or locking desk drawer); and discovering audiovisual equipment is damaged or missing right before class, were examples of things they would have liked to have changed. These issues, while not major deterrents to effective job performance, indicated to the adjunct faculty members that their roles, status, and time demands were less highly regarded than expected. However, they often decided not to express their concerns because the issues appeared too minor and idiosyncratic at the time.

Using the Adjunct Position as a Career Building Block

While working as an adjunct faculty member has several advantages for building a strong career in occupational therapy education, not all future academic endeavors will be achieved through this means. There is little evidence to indicate that academic institutions prefer hiring adjunct faculty from *within* the institution to people outside the institution for full-time faculty appointments (Gappa & Leslie, 1993). Occupational therapy educational programs may operate differently than other academic departments, but there is no data to describe adjunct to full-time hiring practices in OT. Failure to achieve full-time status via an adjunct position is not a direct challenge to the adjunct role per se but may, instead, be a challenge to an adjunct faculty member's long-range career goals.

Culture Shock

Practitioners new to academic settings may experience a work culture different from the practice setting. Compared to professionals in other work settings, faculty members enjoy a high level of autonomy and relative lack of supervision (Fife, 1994). Left on their own to develop course content and materials, some practitioners may interpret the academic freedom so valued by full-time faculty as lack of concern for their work. Socialization into an academic culture is not a one-way process but involves reciprocal interaction among many persons (Crepeau, Thibodaux, & Parham, 1999). Because socialization occurs in multiple ways, the messages conveying the values and beliefs of the organization are open to a variety of interpretations and misinterpretations (Tierney & Rhoads, 1994). Confusion regarding institutional priorities and mores can cause frustration and can hinder work effectiveness.

STRATEGIES FOR SUCCESS AS AN OCCUPATIONAL THERAPY TEACHER-PRACTITIONER

While there are a number of potential challenges to managing the dual roles of adjunct instructor and practitioner, they can be avoided with increased awareness and careful planning. The strategies for success that follow are based on the information obtained in the literature and feedback from occupational therapy teacher-practitioners. Since adjunct faculty roles will vary from one setting to the next, each OT practitioner considering adjunct teaching will have to determine which strategies will work best for her or him.

Initial Negotiations and Skillful Communication

Successful and satisfying adjunct teaching begins with negotiating and understanding the role of the adjunct faculty member in a specific OT department. Direct, proactive communication with the program director demonstrates an applicant's interest in performing the adjunct role well. It is especially important for the applicant along with the program director to determine whether her/his abilities are consistent with the needs and expectations of the teaching position.

Asking thoughtful questions during an interview may be as useful to the program director as it is to the applicant because it may help a program director identify barriers to adjunct faculty development. Since so much about adjunct positions is left to the discretion of the program director, open communication with the person in this role is imperative. A series of meetings may be required during the interview/negotiation process in order to develop a job description that is acceptable to both clinical managers and academic program directors.

Talking with current and past adjunct faculty members may help in developing a list of pertinent questions to ask during the interview process. Questions should be directed toward defining and clarifying the role of the adjunct faculty member. The questions should cover such topics as adjuncts' involvement in committee work and curriculum development, requirements for attending faculty meetings, general departmental operations/daily routines, and availability of physical resources and support personnel to complete teaching-related tasks. The authors also recommend that practitioners applying for adjunct positions use the interview to ask the program director to describe the mission, philosophy, and curriculum design of the department.

During the interview process, it is essential to ask questions that lead to an understanding of what is required to prepare the course (or courses) in question. It is appropriate to ask about required course content and the amount of instructor discretion allowed in course development and management. For example, is it permissible to invite guest lecturers to speak, and, if so, are honoraria available? Is it customary or required to schedule breaks into a class presentation? If the course has been taught before and teaching materials (e.g., previous lecture notes, handouts, or evaluation kits) are available, the applicant can ask to look at them to get a sense of how useful they are and whether they need to be updated. The applicant will probably want to know whether purchasing new equipment for a course is an option and whether there are useful resources available on campus that he/she can have access to. For example, a School of Education in a university may provide information on instructional technologies; computer services may offer test scoring and analysis.

Finally, the applicant will want to ask whether the program director has a sense of the extent and duration of the need for the adjunct faculty role. More specifically, will it be possible to teach the course more than once? A discussion about extent and duration of the adjunct position can provide the applicant with the opportunity to explore long-range potential for adjuncts in the department and to identify areas of interest for future teaching. Academic departments can be rather dynamic, with changes in job responsibilities occurring quickly. Full-time faculty can be temporarily released from teaching responsibilities to complete funded research projects and for maternity leave, illness, or temporary appointment to other university positions. Adjunct faculty members who have expressed interest in other courses and demonstrate flexibility and effective teaching may be able to sustain their employment in a department indefinitely.

Orientation

Receiving a formal orientation to the academic program and having a designated person who is responsible for answering questions about daily operations is essential to success in an adjunct position. An applicant to an adjunct faculty position should determine whether the department has standard procedures for orienting new adjunct faculty and request an orientation to the department, the curriculum, and the course(s) he/she will be teaching. Some academic programs have developed handbooks for adjunct faculty members. If such a handbook is not available, a manual designed for student use may temporarily help to clarify departmental policies and procedures while one for adjunct faculty members is developed.

Optimally, orientation policies and procedures should be developed by the individual responsible for the supervision of adjunct teachers and well understood by the entire faculty. Responsibility for the orientation process can be divided among administrative personnel and faculty. For example, an office manager could answer questions regarding routine tasks such as how to get copies made on time, how to order books and materials for courses, and how to complete forms to get paid. The faculty member supervising the adjunct instructor can cover teaching expectations, curriculum design, and evaluation procedures.

Becoming Socialized into Academia

The values and beliefs of an academic institution are transmitted through explicit and implicit messages (Crepeau, Thibodaux, & Parham, 1999). These messages may be conveyed through formal means (e.g., policies and procedures, ceremonial occasions) or through less formal means (e.g., interaction with others) (Crepeau, Thibodaux, & Parham, 1999). Adjunct faculty should not underestimate the importance of being present at important departmental events (e.g., graduations, thesis defenses), especially if they worked with the students involved. Social activities involving academic co-workers can also provide adjunct faculty members with insights into academic culture and opportunities to build a network of supports to help set priorities. In addition to attending professional conferences and workshops where educational issues are discussed, adjunct faculty members can learn more about academic culture by joining the AOTA Education Special Interest Section (SIS) or the AOTA Education SIS list-serv.

Respectfully Voice Concerns

Adjunct faculty are encouraged to bring the issues that have an impact on teaching effectiveness (e.g., quality of audiovisual equipment, need for a private location to meet with students) to the appropriate party. In many cases, these types of concerns may be more prevalent among the entire faculty than it appears, so teaching peers may be sympathetic and invested in creating solutions. Recognizing that the sum total of a list of seemingly minor annoyances may accumulate into a considerable amount of stress and become a deterrent to good teaching, a program director may be eager to find a remedy if the concerns are brought to her/his attention.

Evaluation and Feedback

The authors recommend that new adjunct teachers request formal feedback from experienced instructors on content of lecture and lab material; teaching methods; organization, effectiveness, and time management in and out of class; test content and methods; grading criteria; availability to students in and out of class; and teacher-student rapport. If a peer review system is not in place in the program, the adjunct faculty member can invite a peer to observe and comment on a class. The adjunct faculty member can gain valuable insights into her/his teaching by letting a peer observer know what specific feedback is being sought and by sharing in advance what will be covered and what teaching methods will be used.

Adjunct faculty should use both formal and informal methods to elicit periodic feedback from students. A formal mid-course evaluation is an effective means of acquiring students' feedback regarding course strengths and limitations. Using customized addenda to standard department evaluation forms to get feedback on specific concerns is also recommended.

While it is important to seek and understand students' input, adjunct faculty must recognize that students will not have all of the insight and experience needed to provide informed input regarding how well a course meets curriculum objectives. Students cannot serve as fully informed consumers of course content, since they are taking the course to become informed. When an adjunct faculty member, especially a relatively new instructor, processes feedback from student evaluations, it may be helpful to reflect on the course with a teaching peer or the program director. Adjunct instructors should try to screen strong reactions, look for honest feedback and consistent themes in students' comments, and use that feedback to improve effectiveness in future teaching and other professional endeavors.

Planning and Managing Time for Teaching

As discussed, teaching requires extensive blocks of preparation time for tasks like preparing lectures and discussions, grading exams, meeting individually with students, and providing feedback on homework assignments. This is especially true for courses that an instructor has never taught before. Teacher-practitioners should expect to spend approximately four out-of-class preparation hours and sometimes more for every hour of in-class time.

It is easier to manage time when one knows in advance the time intensive nature of teaching, but, no matter how skilled one may be at time management, teaching efficiency develops with ongoing experience. Still, books and courses on time management can expedite this process as can getting advice from colleagues who appear to manage their time well.

Another essential time management strategy for an adjunct faculty member is to carefully negotiate with clinical supervisors job responsibilities and necessary release time. Managing two challenging roles (i.e., teacher and practitioner) also requires careful negotiating with peers. With all of these added demands, adjunct faculty may need help to remind themselves that teaching gets easier with time and experience and that the adjunct teaching experience can foster professional development and enhance effectiveness in other areas of practice.

Adjunct Faculty Teaching Salaries

While salary does not usually reflect the hours one has put into developing a course, it is in the best interest of the adjunct faculty member and the department to negotiate a salary that is satisfactory to both. Adjunct faculty members do not typically list salary as a primary reason for seeking teaching positions. However, some adjunct faculty members do emphasize that financial remuneration is an important consideration for accepting adjunct positions and continuing in them. An adjunct faculty member should consider the uniqueness of what he/she is offering the OT department, years of experience as a teacher-practitioner, and the level of responsibility associated with the adjunct position, when discussing salary with a program director.

Sometimes other appealing benefits can be made available to adjunct faculty members to offset an otherwise modest salary. For example, the adjunct faculty member should inquire about tuition reimbursement or departmentally funded continuing education opportunities.

Creating a Network

An active teacher-practitioner moving rapidly between academic and clinical settings may begin to feel isolated and out of touch with what is occurring in both environments. Therefore, it is important to develop a supportive network of both clinical and teaching colleagues. It may be especially helpful to create a network of teacher-practitioners within the local community. Using word of mouth inquiries among occupational therapists, organizing more formal special interest groups via state occupational therapy associations, or creating chat rooms and list-servs on the Internet are some ways of creating networks. Adjunct faculty are also likely to find support among full-time faculty in the occupational therapy program in which they teach. Developing supportive contacts with full-time faculty can lead to a more formal mentoring relationship if desired.

CONCLUSION

Simultaneously teaching in an academic program and providing direct service in an OT practice setting presents special challenges. However, there are also considerable rewards for practitioners who can learn to manage these challenges. Occupational therapy practitioners who become adjunct faculty members make a highly significant contribution to occupational therapy education, gain access to resources for increasing and updating knowledge of particular subject areas, and achieve new and valuable experiences by teaching in academic programs.

The challenges facing adjunct faculty members in academic OT programs include job and status insecurity, unmet evaluation and orientation needs, and the added stress of working in more than one environment. However, the adjunct faculty members who were interviewed did not regard these challenges as insurmountable. In fact, several praised occupational therapy departments for highly professional and innovative ways of meeting challenges and exceeding their expectations.

By making use of the proposed strategies for success in adjunct faculty positions, individual adjunct faculty members and the occupational therapy programs in which they teach can develop a collaborative process of minimizing challenges and maximizing benefits. Carefully designing individual adjunct faculty roles that meet the needs of adjuncts, students, and faculty in an occupational therapy program is a key factor in assuring the success of adjunct faculty members. There is no reason to assume that interested adjunct faculty cannot or will not accept and welcome responsibilities beyond teaching. Some of the teacher-practitioners the authors talked with indicated that they willingly served on committees, participated in peer teaching reviews, advised students, and participated in research projects.

Both academic and clinical OT programs can benefit from having teacher-practitioners on staff. Adjunct faculty can provide clinical peers with current information on theory application, newly identified practice guidelines, OT outcome research, faculty research interests, and educational program development trends. The adjunct faculty member can inform academic faculty of current practice trends and the needs of occupational therapists working in a variety of practice settings. By providing such information, adjunct faculty may serve as a bridge to effective communication between practitioners in the community and full-time OT faculty.

Because their experience with direct care is current, adjunct faculty can discuss practice issues from a case-based perspective, incorporating treatment ideas from clients for whom they are providing OT services. They can use up-to-date examples to demonstrate current evaluation and treatment procedures and context-specific clinical reasoning processes for students. For these reasons, employing adjunct faculty may be preferred over graduate student assistants for teaching full courses or conducting labs. While teaching assistantships are frequently available in other academic disciplines, occupational therapy programs, especially those not offering post-professional training, may have fewer graduate students available for teaching assistance. Stronger alliances with the OT practice community, current, case-based teaching, and enhancement of practitioners' skills can be the result of having adjunct faculty in academic occupational therapy programs.

REFERENCES

American Occupational Therapy Association (1997). *Educational Data Survey Report.*
Brayley, C.B. (1996). *From clinician to academician: A handbook for those who aspire to become faculty members.* Bethesda: AOTA.
Crepeau, E.B., Thibodaux, L., & Parham, D. (1999). Academic juggling act: Beginning and sustaining an academic career. *The American Journal of Occupational Therapy, 53,* 25-30.

Fife, J.D. (1994). Foreword. In W.G. Tierney & R.A. Rhoads (Eds.), *Faculty social-ization as cultural process: A mirror of institutional commitment* (pp. xiii-xiv). ASHE-ERIC Higher Education Report no. 93-6. Washington, DC: George Washington University, School of Education and Human Development.

Gappa, J.M., & Leslie, D.W. (1993). *The invisible faculty: Improving the status of part timers in higher education.* San Francisco: Jossey-Bass Inc., Publishers.

Johnson, J.A. (1978). Issues in education. *The American Journal of Occupational Therapy, 32,* 355-358.

Leatherman, C. (1997). Do accreditors look the other way when colleges rely on part-timers? *The Chronicle of Higher Education,* November.

Parham, D. (1985). Award structures and occupational therapy faculty. Part II: Predictors of rewards and scholarly activity. *Occupational Therapy Journal of Research, 5,* 83-100.

Parham, D. (1987). Brief: The perceived impact of research on the activities and evaluation of occupational therapy faculty. *Occupational Therapy Journal of Research, 7,* 126-128.

Rhoades, G. (1996). Reorganizing the faculty workforce for flexibility. *Journal of Higher Education, 67,* 627-657.

Tierney, W.G., & Rhoads, R.A. (1994). *Faculty socialization and cultural process: A mirror of educational commitment.* ASHE-ERIC Higher Education Report No 93-6. Washington, DC: George Washington University, School of Education and Human Development.

Tuckman, H.P. (1978). Who is part-time in academe? *AAUP Bulletin, 64,* 305-315.

STUDENT DEVELOPMENT

Occupational Therapy Students' Learning Styles and Application to Professional Academic Training

Victoria Moji Titiloye, PhD, OTR, RN
Anne Hiller Scott, PhD, OTR, FAOTA

SUMMARY. Methods of optimizing students' learning have been a major concern of educators over time. If occupational therapy educators know the students' learning styles at the onset of their training, teaching can be designed to enhance students' optimal learning throughout their education. This study determined learning styles of 201 junior students (age range = 18-57, mean age = 30.9), enrolled in an urban occupational

Victoria Moji Titiloye is Assistant Professor, Downstate Medical Center, Occupational Therapy Program, Brooklyn, NY 11203.

Anne Hiller Scott is Program Director, Division of Occupational Therapy, Long Island University Brooklyn Campus, 1 University Plaza, Brooklyn, NY 11201.

Address correspondence to: Victoria Titiloye, Assistant Professor, Downstate Medical Center, Occupational Therapy Program, 450 Clarkson Avenue, Box 81, Brooklyn, NY 11203.

[Haworth co-indexing entry note]: "Occupational Therapy Students' Learning Styles and Application to Professional Academic Training." Titiloye, Victoria Moji, and Anne Hiller Scott. Co-published simultaneously in *Occupational Therapy in Health Care* (The Haworth Press, Inc.) Vol. 15, No. 1/2, 2001, pp. 145-155; and: *Education for Occupational Therapy in Health Care: Strategies for the New Millennium* (eds: Patricia Crist, and Marjorie Scaffa) The Haworth Press, Inc., 2001, pp. 145-155. Single or multiple copies of this article are available for a fee from The Haworth Document Delivery Service [1-800-HAWORTH, 9:00 a.m. - 5:00 p.m. (EST). E-mail address: getinfo@haworthpressinc.com].

therapy program from 1990 to 1999. Kolb's Learning Style Inventory, a 12-item questionnaire, was administered to the students in the spring of their junior years. Their learning styles were determined using Kolb's criteria. Results yielded: variations in students' preferred learning styles in each class from year to year; higher percentage of convergers (mean = 35%), fewer divergers (mean = 18%). Overall, students were mostly convergers (mean = 35%) and assimilators (mean = 25%). Applications of the findings to teaching students are discussed. *[Article copies available for a fee from The Haworth Document Delivery Service: 1-800-HAWORTH. E-mail address: <getinfo@haworthpressinc.com> Website: <http://www.HaworthPress.com>* © 2001 by The Haworth Press, Inc. All rights reserved.]*

KEYWORDS. Learning styles, education, allied health students

INTRODUCTION

Methods of enhancing students' optimal learning have been a major concern of educators for some time (Laschinger, 1984; Dunn and Dunn, 1978; Keefe, 1982). Many theories and models have been developed to better understand processes of learning (De Bello, 1990; Gregorc, 1985a, 1985b; Kolb, 1981; Dunn and Dunn, 1978). Learning is a method used to adapt to and cope with the world around us. People learn differently. We each develop a preferred learning style based on our unique set of experiences (Kolb, 1981; Kolb, 1984). Learning styles are the ways we prefer to absorb and incorporate new information.

Learning style affects how we solve problems, make decisions, and develop and change our attitudes and behavior (Kolb, 1984). Theories suggest that individuals learn optimally when they are taught in their preferred learning style. Therefore, if educators know students' preferred learning styles, teaching can be designed to meet the learning needs of the students at the onset of their training, thereby enhancing optimal learning throughout their training period. To date, there is limited information available on the predominant learning style of Occupational Therapy students; hence, this study was performed.

LEARNING STYLE LITERATURE

Many learning models have been developed (Gregorc, 1985a, 1985b; Kolb, 1981; Dunn and Dunn, 1978). Kolb's experiential learning theory is most commonly applied by health care professions (Farina, 1998; Katz and Heimann, 1991; Laschinger, 1984). The core of the theory is the description of the learning cycle. The cycle emphasizes how experience is translated into concepts, which, in turn, are used as guides in choice of new experiences. The theory states that learning involves a four stage cycle, namely concrete experience, reflective observation, abstract conceptualization, and active experimentation. Concrete experience forms the basis for observations and reflections. Observations and reflections are, in turn, assimilated and distilled into theory or concepts from which new implications for actions can be drawn.

The concrete experience stage emphasizes feeling as opposed to thinking. It focuses on dealing with immediate human situations in a personal way and learning occurs through feeling. The reflective observation stage focuses on understanding the meaning of ideas and situations through careful observation, and learning occurs by watching. The abstract conceptualization stage focuses on use of logic, ideas, and concepts. It emphasizes thinking and learning occurs by doing. The active experimentation stage emphasizes practical applications as opposed to feeling. Each stage in the cycle is referred to as learning mode, and for an individual to learn effectively, one has to be able to adapt to and apply the skills in each of the four learning modes (Kolb and Smith, 1986).

There is variation on individuals' reliance on a particular learning mode. One's learning style is predicated on which learning modes an individual predominantly utilizes. Kolb identified four learning styles: divergers, assimilators, convergers, and accommodators (Kolb, 1984; Kolb and Smith, 1986). Convergers' dominant learning abilities are abstract conceptualization and active experimentation. Convergers can focus on specific problems through deductive reasoning. They are strong in problem solving, decision making, and application of theories. They prefer dealing with technical tasks and problems. Divergers are strong in reflective observation and concrete experience. They view concrete situations from many perspectives, and are best in situations that demand generation of alternative ideas and implications. Divergers are interested in people, and their strengths include imaginative abilities, awareness of meaning and values. They perform better in situations that require generation of alternative ideas and brainstorming, and learn best when content is presented to them in different ways. Assimilators utilize reflective observation and abstract conceptualization modes. Assimilators are concerned with ideas and abstract concepts, and are good at assimilating disparate observations into integrated explanations. Assimilators are strongest in inductive reasoning and the ability to create theoretical models. In contrast, accommodators' learning abilities are in active experimentation with what is to be learned. They utilize active experimentation and concrete experience modes. Accommodators are best suited for situations that require one to adapt to changing immediate circumstances. They are strongest in doing things, taking risks, and engaging in new experiences. They achieve best when given the opportunity to learn by actively engaging and trying out that which is to be learned, and by problem solving through trial and error (Kolb, 1984; Kolb and Smith, 1986). Strengths of convergers are opposite those of divergers. Similarly, the strengths of assimilators are opposite those of accommodators (Kolb, 1984).

Kolb (1984) indicated that no one learning environment is oriented towards just one learning style, but rather a combination of behavioral and affective learning environments yields a work setting climate. An individual may reject and/or resist learning environments that are dissimilar to the person's preferred learning style (Kolb 1984). Kolb (1984) maintains that career choice and learning style relate to one another. Kolb and Wolfe (1981) proposed that the structure and nature of different professions create an environmental press which requires a learner to use particular learning abilities and competencies. Kolb contends that human service professions have people with concrete learning styles. Research has demonstrated distinctive profiles for different professions.

A few studies have found that the nursing profession attracts more accommodators and divergers (Rakoczy and Money, 1995; Laschinger, 1986; Laschinger and Boss, 1983). A study conducted on physical therapy students, from programs in three different countries, reported convergent and assimilative learning styles to be predominant (Farina, 1998). Katz and Heimann (1991) determined the learning styles of five groups of Israeli health professions students and practitioners. Their results indicated that occupational therapy students were more concrete, as compared to those in clinical psychology, nursing, physical therapy, and social work. Katz and Heimann (1991) also noted that all four health professions, excluding psychology, emphasized active learning rather than reflective learning (associated with divergers) and that concrete orientation was higher for all first-year students. Occupational therapists and students were accommodators; clinical psychology, social work, and nursing students were divergers. Physical therapy students were convergers, with practitioners being assimilators who were close to the border of divergers. Social work practitioners were accommodators while nurses were convergers. The authors suggested that occupational therapy educators need to find ways to integrate conceptual work into a student's active learning style. Katz (1990) tested the hypothesis that students would perform better when matched for learning style and appropriate teaching method than those for whom teaching and learning conditions were mismatched. Reflective students required less time to learn material when they were exposed to lectures and the opposite was true for active students.

DESCRIPTION OF THE PARTICIPANTS

Two hundred and one occupational therapy juniors in an accredited two-and-a-half year upper division program in an urban setting participated in this study. The sample was comprised of students in their junior years from 1990 to 1999. An average of 20 students participated each year within the 10-year period. They ranged in age from 18 to 57 years (mean = 30.9 years). They had completed 12 science courses, five occupational therapy courses, and were at the end of their first academic year in the program at the time of the study. Six female faculty members with teaching experience ranging from 5-21 years also participated in the study. The faculty were selected to determine if their learning style matched that of the majority of students.

DATA COLLECTION PROCEDURE

The Kolb LSI was given to the students during a class period in their junior years by one member of the faculty. A cover letter explaining the purpose of the study was attached to the LSI, and students were asked to read it before completing the LSI. Participation was voluntary. They were informed that they had a choice not to participate. The Kolb LSI is a 12-item Likert scale questionnaire. For each item, students were required to rate themselves on a scale of 4-1, selecting the answer that best describes the way they learn (rating scale: 4 = Most like you, 3 = Second most like you, 2 = Third most like you, 1 = Least like you). The Kolb LSI identifies four learning styles: convergers, divergers, assimilators, and accommodators (Kolb, 1984; Kolb and Smith, 1986).

The LSI is reported to be very reliable, with an alpha reliability coefficient range of 0.76 to 0.91 (Kolb and Smith, 1986). Its validity was determined by factor analysis procedures which extracted only three of Kolb's four factors (Bourguignon, 1994). The Kolb LSI is one of the most commonly used learning style inventories by health care professionals (De Bello, 1990).

DATA ANALYSIS

Responses for each participant were scored using directions in the Kolb LSI manual (Kolb, 1976). Each student's dominant learning style and learning modes were determined using the scoring calculations specified in Kolb's manual (Kolb, 1976; Kolb and Smith, 1986). Then the percentage of the number of students with the respective learning styles described by Kolb, namely, divergers, convergers, accommodators, and assimilators, was calculated for each year. The two most common learning styles preferred by the group as a whole were determined.

FINDINGS

Results yielded variations in subjects' preferred learning styles in each class from year to year (see Table 1). Figure 1 depicts the variation in the percentage of students' learning styles in 1991 and 1999. Overall there was a higher percentage of convergers and fewer divergers. Cumulative data showed that convergers ranged from 10%-60% with a mean of 36% (see Table 1). The percentage of divergers ranged from 0%-29% with a mean of 18% (see Table 1). Assimilators ranged from 15%-40% (mean = 25%) while accommodators had a range of 8%-40% with a mean of 21% (see Table 1). There was a shift in the percentage of convergers (mean = 25%) in the first five years (1990 to 1994) compared to that (mean = 44%) of the last five years (1995 to 1999). Four of the faculty members were convergers while two were assimilators.

DISCUSSION

Findings from our study indicate that the learning styles of occupational therapy students in this study are similar to those reported for physical therapists (Farina, 1998), a field closely related to occupational therapy, with similar requirements for admission. Contrarily, Katz and Heimann (1991) found Israeli occupational therapy students in her study to be more concrete than those in other health professions. This variation reported may be due to cultural differences in the educational environment and admission requirements. As stated by Kolb (1984), affective and behavioral demands of the learning environment may require different learning competencies from the students. The most common preferred learning styles in this cohort of students were convergers and assimilators. Both physical and occupational therapy professions require detailed analysis and synthesis of information, arriving at objective, verifiable decisions and judgments. The students' education and training requires them to analyze and synthesize both didactic and clinical observation in an objective manner and arrive at a logical rationale for selecting specific treatment approaches to client care. According to Kolb's learning model, all these skills are strengths of convergers and assimilators. In addition, faculty members' preferred learning styles match those of the majority of the students.

TABLE 1. Percentage of Students with Each Learning Style in Each Class from 1990 (Year 1) to 1999 (Year 10)

	Converger	Diverger	Assimilator	Accommodator
1990	29%	25%	21%	25%
1991	10%	29%	38%	24%
1992	33%	28%	22%	17%
1993	29%	20%	29%	20%
1994	26%	22%	40%	13%
1995	50%	25%	17%	8%
1996	32%	16%	32%	16%
1997	45%	0%	16%	40%
1998	33%	7%	15%	37%
1999	60%	5%	22%	12%
Mean	35%	18%	25%	21%

By contrast, nursing students have been found to be mostly accommodators and divergers (Rakoczy and Money, 1995). The nurse's role entails making decisions quickly and moving into action to effect treatment, which is one of the strengths of accommodators. People seem to be attracted to careers that require their learning needs/characteristics (Kolb, 1984). Though there was a higher percentage of convergers in this OT cohort, a notable shift occurred in the percentage of convergers in the first five years, compared with the last five years. This might be due to the fact that there were more mature students and second career students admitted. These students tend to be clearer about their goals and the requirements of the programs and, therefore, more accurate in matching the needs of the program with their strengths. Also our program has a reputation for being very strong in the sciences and may tend to attract more students with the convergent learning style.

Teaching students in their preferred learning style and matching teaching techniques and methods to students' learning styles will enhance students' optimal learning and retention. Literature reveals that when there are incongruencies be-

FIGURE 1. Comparison of Students' Learning Styles in 1991 and 1999

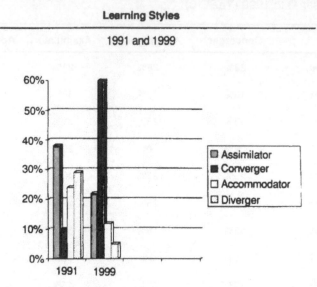

tween students' learning styles and teachers' teaching techniques and learning styles, students performed significantly lower (scored in the C-range grade) as compared to when students' learning styles matched those of the faculty (Joyce-Nagata, 1996; Hughes, Atkinson, and Williams, 1993). This further supports the findings from studies indicating that when students learn in their preferred learning styles and teachers' techniques meet the diversified learning style needs of the students, the students perform better (Nelson, Dunn, and Griggs, 1993).

DIRECT APPLICATION OF STUDY'S FINDINGS TO PROFESSIONAL PREPARATION

Though the students mostly prefer convergent and assimilative learning styles, the clients that they will be treating in the clinical settings may learn best in other learning styles. The findings of this study were applied to students' professional training in two ways. First, the students were taught how to determine their own most and least preferred learning styles with the Kolb LSI. Then students learned about the strengths and preferred learning situations for themselves and also learned about each of Kolb's other three learning styles. Second, this was followed by assignments that challenged them to teach an activity a colleague is interested in learning. The student teacher is required to identify his or her least preferred learning style and teach a colleague in that learning style. The emphasis is on the student teacher's teaching style. This assignment attempts to simulate what the student is likely to encounter in a real clinical situation when a client with a different learning style may be in the student's care and needs to be taught in the best way he/she can most benefit from the therapeutic process. As part of the assignment, the student teacher is required to set measurable goals on how he/she will set up the teaching in a way to optimize learning for an individual whose most preferred learning is the student teacher's least utilized learning style.

Students have reported that these assignments encourage them to view learning from the learner's point of view rather than just from their's alone. They reported that the experience allows them to plan their teaching better and requires them to think and incorporate material, cues, and techniques that will facilitate their teaching-learning interactions and develop creative ways in teaching other people so that learning can best occur. For example, some students who are accommodators and who utilize the convergent learning style the least had to teach their colleagues who are convergers. Accommodators learn best by trial and error and directly doing things. Convergers, on the other hand, learn best by logically following a step-by-step procedure, reading instructions or handouts or diagrams. The student teacher who is an accommodator had to seek out information on the optimal ways a converger learns, then develop a step-by-step instruction on how the task to be taught is performed as well as find or draw out sequences of the performance to guide the learner. At the end, the student teacher is also required to assess the colleagues' learning and obtain feedback on whether the teaching techniques facilitated learning or impeded it.

Faculty members have also used the knowledge of students' learning styles in each class to design their teaching to meet the learning needs of each student. This includes designing practical learning situations and assignments, setting up student discussion groups and fieldwork assignments. Though the faculty are convergers and assimilators, they still have to facilitate optimal learning in students with different preferred learning styles. For fieldwork assignments, as much as possible, attempts are made to match students with clinical supervisors and settings that may be optimal for the students' learning styles and needs. Our faculty fieldwork coordinator communicates frequently with site supervisors and learns about their strengths, the learning environment, and work load expectations for students. This information is then utilized to match the students to the sites. Students are given information and suggestions about fieldwork sites that may optimally facilitate their learning. Also, seminars have been held for fieldwork supervisors, both in our program and in their respective clinical settings, on the application of learning styles to students' fieldwork training. Kolb's learning model's characteristics and learning styles are discussed, and optimal learning situations for students with each learning style are shared. Supervisors are encouraged to apply what they have learned about learning styles and optimal learning situations to their teaching-learning interaction with the students and also to ask for help if they need further guidance in applying what they have learned to the students' fieldwork supervision. Though this study has direct application, more studies are needed to determine the effectiveness of applying the knowledge of learning style to all aspects of OT education.

REFERENCES

Bourguignon, C. M. (1994). *Application of the thinking-feeling-acting behavior model to learning of baccalaureate student nurses.* University of Toledo.

De Bello, C. T. (1990). Comparison of eleven major learning styles models: Variables, appropriate populations, validity of instrumentation, and the research behind them. *Reading, Writing, and Learning Disabilities, 6*: 203-222.

Dunn, R., and Dunn, K. (1978). *Teaching students through their individual learning styles.* Englewood Cliffs, NJ: Prentice Hall, Inc.

Farina, N. J. (1998). How do physical therapy students learn? Applicability of Briggs and Kolb's learning models to physical therapy students in three countries. *Physical Therapy, 78* (5): S 53.

Gregorc, A. F. (1985a). *Inside styles: Beyond the basics.* Columbis, CT: Gregorc Associates Inc.

Gregorc, A. F. (1985b). *Style delineator.* Maynard, MA: Gabriel Systems.

Hughes, R. B., Atkinson, G., Jr., and Williams, C. L. (1993). Success in baccalaureate nursing programs: A matter of accommodation? *Journal of Nursing Education, 32* (2): 64-70.

Joyce-Nagata, B. (1996). Students' academic performance in nursing as a function of student and faculty congruency. *Journal of Nursing Education, 25* (9): 366-371.

Katz, N., and Heimann, N. (1991). Learning style of students and practitioners in five health professions. *Occupational Therapy Journal of Research, 11* (4): 238-244.

Katz, N. (1990). Problem solving and time: Functions of learning style and teaching methods. *Occupational Therapy Journal of Research, 10* (4): 221-236.

Keefe, J. W. (1982). Assessing student learning styles. In Keefe, J. W. (Ed.), *Student learning styles and brain behavior* (pp. 1-18). Reston, VA: National Association of Secondary Schools Principals.

Kolb, D. A. (1976). *Learning Style Inventory and technical manual.* Boston, MA: McBer.

Kolb, D. A. (1981). Experiential learning and the learning style inventory. A response to Friedman and Stumpf. *Academic Management Review, 6* (2): 289-296.

Kolb, D. A. (1984). *Experiential learning. Experience the source of learning and development.* Englewood Cliffs, NJ: Prentice Hall, Inc.

Kolb, D.A., and Wolfe, D. (1981). *Professional education and career development. A cross-sectional study of adaptive competencies in experiential learning.* Cleveland, OH: Case Western Reserve University.

Kolb, D. A., and Smith, A. M. (1986). *User's guide for the Learning Style Inventory. A manual for teachers and trainers.* Boston, MA: McBer and Company.

Laschinger, H. K., and Boss, M. (1983). Learning styles of nursing students and career choice. *Journal of Advanced Nursing,* 9: 375-380.

Laschinger, H. K. (1984). Learning styles of nursing students and career choices. *Journal of Advances in Nursing, 84* (9): 735-780.

Laschinger, H. K. (1986). Learning styles of nursing students and environmental press perceptions of two clinical nursing settings. *Journal of Advanced Nursing,* 11: 289-294.

Nelson, B., Dunn, R., and Griggs, S. A. (1993). Effects of learning style intervention on students' achievement and retention. *Journal of College Student Development, 34:* 364-369.

Rakoczy, M., and Money, S. (1995). Learning styles of nursing students: A 3-year cohort longitudinal study. *Journal of Professional Nursing,* 11, 170-174.

Educating Scholars of Practice: An Approach to Preparing Tomorrow's Researchers

Joy Hammel, PhD, OTR/L, FAOTA
Marcia Finlayson, PhD, OT(C), OTR/L
Gary Kielhofner, Dr. PH, OTR/L, FAOTA
Christine A. Helfrich, PhD, OTR/L
Elizabeth Peterson, MPH, OTR/L

SUMMARY. Occupational therapy's scholarship too often fails to result in a cumulative body of knowledge that is directly relevant to practice, and links theory and research to practice. This problem has its basis in how therapists are prepared to make scholarly contributions to the field. This article describes an educational strategy for preparing scholars of practice whose work will contribute to building a knowledge base that examines and enhances practice. The strategy is based upon social learning theory, employs principles of situated learning and cognitive apprenticeship, and involves students as members of an ongoing community of

Joy Hammel is Assistant Professor, Marcia Finlayson is Assistant Professor, Gary Kielhofner is Head and Professor, Christine A. Helfrich is Assistant Professor, and Elizabeth Peterson is Clinical Assistant Professor, all affiliated with the University of Illinois at Chicago, Department of Occupational Therapy, 1919 W. Taylor Street, MC 811, Chicago, IL 60612.

The authors would like to acknowledge the faculty, students, staff, visiting scholars, and community collaborators involved in the development and implementation of the Scholarship of Practice at the University of Illinois at Chicago.

[Haworth co-indexing entry note]: "Educating Scholars of Practice: An Approach to Preparing Tomorrow's Researchers." Hammel, Joy et al. Co-published simultaneously in *Occupational Therapy in Health Care* (The Haworth Press, Inc.) Vol. 15, No. 1/2, 2001, pp. 157-176; and: *Education for Occupational Therapy in Health Care: Strategies for the New Millennium* (eds: Patricia Crist, and Marjorie Scaffa) The Haworth Press, Inc., 2001, pp. 157-176. Single or multiple copies of this article are available for a fee from The Haworth Document Delivery Service [1-800-HAWORTH, 9:00 a.m. - 5:00 p.m. (EST). E-mail address: getinfo@haworthpressinc.com].

scholars. Steps to and benefits of creating this scholarly community and implementing this educational strategy are discussed. *[Article copies available for a fee from The Haworth Document Delivery Service: 1-800-HAWORTH. E-mail address: <getinfo@haworthpressinc.com> Website: <http://www.HaworthPress.com> © 2001 by The Haworth Press, Inc. All rights reserved.]*

KEYWORDS. Graduate education, mentoring, social learning theory, applied research

INTRODUCTION

Writing in the *Chronicle of Higher Education*, sociologist Theodore Kemper (2000) recently decried the failure of sociology to develop a science that offers substantial, empirically grounded insights into the nature of society. As symptom of the field's failure to garner a cumulative body of knowledge, he pointed to a recent meeting of the American Sociological Association in which "no two papers dealt with the same problem in a focused, solution-oriented way" (p. 1). While Kemper's observation might be overstated, his point is readily transposed to characterize occupational therapy's professional meetings and, by extension, its literature. In fact, the observation made two decades ago by Christiansen (1981) that occupational therapy lacked cumulative scholarship is, to an unsettling extent, still accurate today.

Occupational therapy literature is prone to serve up papers espousing a set of ideas whose differences from prior published work, including work from outside the profession, can be questioned. At the same time, there are far less examples of empirical work that clearly contribute to and build upon an established line of research, and a substantive body of knowledge, over time. Hence, Kemper's (2000) observation that sociologists have a "distressingly low regard for cumulative knowledge" (p. 2) and "prize originality to a fault" (p. 2) could also be taken as accurate descriptions of occupational therapy scholarship.

Occupational therapy's status as an applied discipline raises a further, though related, problem. While there is clearly a growing body of theoretical concepts being articulated in the field (e.g., Dunn, Brown & McGuigan, 1994; Kielhofner, 1995; Law, Cooper, Strong, Stewart, Rigby & Letts, 1996; Townsend, 1997; Nelson, 1986; Schkade & Schultz, 1992; Schultz & Schkade, 1992; Zemke & Clark, 1996), there is a parallel disillusionment on the part of practitioners about the relevance of these concepts to practice (Hammel, 2000; Kielhofner, 2000). There is also a lack of consistent connections between the research being done and the practical concerns of therapists and of the communities they serve (Abreu, Peloquin & Ottenbacher, 1998). Consequently, there is a significant gap between knowledge generated in academia and the need for knowledge in everyday practice.

In response to this state of affairs, we have sought at the University of Illinois (UIC) to educate new scholars in a way that prepares them to contribute to the development of a cumulative body of empirically tested and practically applied knowledge. Consistent with Kennedy's (1997) view of scholarship and the responsibilities of academicians, we organize our training of future scholars around the following elements:

1. Designing, conducting, and disseminating research that contributes to practice;
2. Negotiating and building partnerships with individuals and organizations outside of the academic department to create new educational, practice and research opportunities; and
3. Creating an intellectual environment that results in synergies to advance the practice and scholarship of occupational therapy, and to make an active contribution to related bodies of knowledge.

The purpose of this article is to describe our approach to teaching scholarship and creating a community of scholarship for faculty, students, and community collaborators. We will explain the steps we have taken and the challenges we have faced as we have operationalized this approach. Finally, we will describe the faculty productivity, student learning, and community building outcomes of our efforts.

AN APPROACH TO TEACHING SCHOLARSHIP

Our approach to teaching scholarship is based upon social learning theory (Vygotsky, 1978) and operationalized through the use of a situated learning approach (Anderson, Reder & Simon, 1996; Lave & Wenger, 1991; Stein, 1998; Wilson, 1993) and cognitive apprenticeships (Berryman, 1990; Collins, Brown & Newman, 1989; Collins, 1991; Lave, 1988). The basic tenet of social learning theory is that learning is cultivated through immersion in practical issues within a social community, and knowledge is acquired and generalized when learned within the context from which it emerges (Brown, Collins & Duguid, 1989). The application of social learning theory creates an environment in which students learn to apply knowledge in context, rather than to reiterate decontextualized information such as that found in a "how to" research text (Kirschner & Whitson, 1997; Willemsen & Gainen, 1995). Both situated learning and cognitive apprenticeship help students link theory, research, and practice (Berryman, 1990; Lieberman, 1993).

Situated learning centers knowledge and skill development within everyday situations. It is based upon the premises that (a) knowledge is acquired and needs to be learned in context, (b) learning results from social processes that involve collaborative problem solving around specific issues, and (c) learning should not be separated from the world of social action and its rich complexity of actors, actions, and situations, which can be catalysts for applied research (Anderson et al., 1996; Lave, 1997; Wilson, 1993). The success of situated learning is dependent upon a *community of practice* to serve as the learning context (Brown, 1994; Lave & Wenger, 1991). Thus, learning becomes a social process embedded in a community of scholars working collaboratively on meaningful issues.

Cognitive apprenticeship (Brown et al., 1989; Collins, Brown & Newman, 1989; Collins, 1991) is a social learning strategy that includes:

1. Learning declarative, procedural, and conditional reasoning in the context of practice;
2. Exploration and risk taking in a context that supports, yet challenges the learner to take on new roles;
3. Modeling and coaching by mentors, followed by realistic, authentic opportunities to practice and immerse into everyday problems and issues; and
4. Reflection and critical analysis of the processes and outcomes learned within a community of practice.

Cognitive apprenticeships are based upon the concept that novices learn first-hand through "doing." Apprentices are immersed in a realistic context and engage in progressively more challenging activities with mentors whom they can observe and challenge (Brown et al., 1989; Lave, 1988; Lave & Wenger, 1991).

In our case, the apprenticeship involves students across the entry-level professional, advanced master, and doctoral levels directly "doing applied scholarship." Instead of learning scholarship primarily through books and lectures, or through projects students undertake alone, we create an environment in which students immerse into scholarship within a social context. When working as apprentices, students learn not only from their advisor or instructors but also from a community of scholars that includes student peers, other faculty, staff, clients, practitioners, and community members involved in the scholarship. All are part of the social learning context, and students learn to flexibly negotiate teacher-learner roles within this community (Lieberman, 1993).

Faculty who are in the position of structuring situated learning opportunities and cognitive apprenticeships must have accomplished themselves what students are to learn. This means that if faculty are to effectively educate students about scholarship, they must be actively engaged in a program of research themselves. Teaching by example is unavoidable when social learning theory is the foundation for teaching scholarship. By extension, students learn scholarship best within a community of scholars building upon each other's work. Consequently, much of our efforts to operationalize our approach to teaching scholarship involves creating a robust, scholarly community. The other strategies aim to make students active participants in this community.

The success of social learning theory hinges on the quality of the learning context. In the sections that follow we describe a series of steps that are supporting the ongoing development and improvement of a scholarly community and its use as a learning context (see Table 1 for a summary).

STEPS TOWARD OPERATIONALIZING THE APPROACH

Step #1: Defining a Common Vision of Departmental Scholarship

A robust community of scholarship requires that members pursue complementary lines of investigation and take advantage of each other's knowledge and expertise. Although individual interests are critical, a set of common themes must pull the scholarship of a department together into a cohesive community. These themes may be substantive and/or methodological, but must facilitate sharing ideas, information, and know-how to advance all participants' scholarship. At UIC, we began the process of defining a common vision of departmental scholarship by searching for common themes in our research. In addition, we considered two unique features of our academic institution: the department's historical mission and our university's identity.

Our department was founded under the vision that the teaching and practice missions should be integrated. A natural extension of this idea was the synthesis of scholarship and practice. UIC's institutional mission focuses on seeking solutions to the economic, cultural, political, and health problems faced by people and organizations within the urban context. This means that the university values and supports those who engage in applied scholarship. Consequently, it was natural for us to develop a program of research tied to practice. The outcome of this process was a document, entitled "A Scholarship of Practice," that clearly defined the common vision of the department's scholarship

TABLE 1. Summary of the Steps and Activities Involved in Achieving a Scholarship of Practice and Creating a Supportive Community of Learning Based on Social Learning Theory

Steps	Activities
Define a common vision of scholarship	• Identify themes of scholarship that reflect department and university mission and identity • Identify community and practice issues that match program themes and mission
Develop and build traditions of scholarship	• Create and document program and faculty long term research plans, including traditions of inquiry • Build communities of faculty, staff, and students working within traditions • Organize student independent studies, research assistantships, experiential activities, and apprentice activities around traditions • Establish community partnerships to support traditions • Develop relationships with scholars from other departments and the community to support research traditions • Develop and implement plans to pursue extramural research funding in identified areas
Make a culture of scholarly collaboration normative	• Provide multiple forums for sharing scholarly activities (e.g., colloquia, seminars, student thesis/project presentations) • Define and negotiate roles and expectations of all members in the community • Develop and maintain clear ground rules for scholarly activities • Identify win-win outcomes of participation in scholarly activities and negotiate plan of action to ensure successful completion
Create research, teaching, and service synergies	• Share and disseminate scholarship with practitioners and the community • Work with selected community sites to collaborate on multiple goals and activities addressing program development, student training, and research simultaneously • Integrate scholarly activities throughout required coursework • Identify collaborative grant, research, and training activities, publication and presentation opportunities
Create vehicles for idea development and constructive commentary	• Provide multiple opportunities for critiquing individual and community scholarship for students, faculty, and community (e.g., writing groups, grant writing, and review groups) • Invite scholars from within and outside the university to share their research activities and to critique scholarship • Implement ongoing mechanisms for the community to create, evaluate, and shape collaborative scholarship activities

(http://www.uic.edu/ahp/OT/grada.htm). The scholarship of practice is envisioned as a dialectic in which theoretical and empirical knowledge is brought to bear on the practical problems and upon which questions are raised and addressed through scholarship (see Figure 1). While research within the scholarship of practice is broad, it is bound together by a common theme: the quest to better understand the needs of people whom occupational therapy serves, and the ways in which we can most effectively address these needs. Our scholar-

FIGURE 1. Dialectic of a Scholarship of Practice in Which Theory, Research, and Practice Consistently Inform and Build upon Each Other Within a Tradition of Inquiry, and Are Integrated Within a Social Learning Community

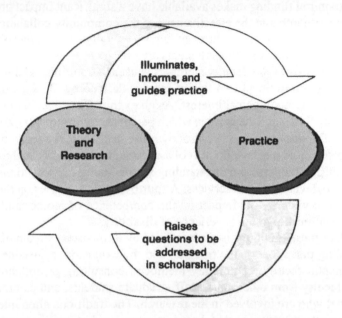

ship of practice further reflects the university's vision to create knowledge relevant to an urban mission, and the profession's commitment to shaping occupation-based practice.

Step #2: Developing and Building Traditions of Inquiry

Conducting research of a high quality follows a developmental process (Case-Smith, 1999) in which a variety of research strategies are integrated over time into a program of research. Some key elements of this process are building theoretical arguments, refining methodological approaches, establishing a track record in a defined substantive content or methodological area, developing relationships with research collaborators and sites, and, most important, securing extramural or external funding to support the research over time.

A limited number of scholars in occupational therapy reach the level of sophistication that enables them to successfully compete for substantial federal and/or private funding to support their research. Yet, in interdisciplinary circles, extramural funding stands as one of the hallmarks of the sophistication, depth, and breadth of one's research program. Certainly, the kinds of resources that extramural funding makes available have a significant impact on the quality of the research and the effectiveness of the community collaboration.

While the concept of a tradition of inquiry encompasses a range of efforts in our department, the following elements are considered basic to each tradition. Ordinarily, two or more faculty members lead each tradition and thus maintain an ongoing commitment to a line of inquiry defined by theoretical, substantive, and/or methodological interest. As an example, one tradition focuses on community living and the ways in which personal, environmental, and societal factors influence choice and control over life decisions. A second tradition is organized around the development of assessments for practice and research. A third tradition focuses on understanding factors that affect vocational success in order to develop related services. A fourth tradition focuses on the problem of domestic violence, its impact on the competence of mother and children, and its relationship to the experience of disability.

Each of these traditions is characterized by a consistent stream of extramural funding that supports the research and, by extension, a sustained team of departmental faculty, community members, consulting or collaborating research faculty from other units, staff, graduate students, and external agency personnel who are involved in the research. The traditions often intersect and complement each other so that there is a natural and mutually supportive relationship between them. These traditions of inquiry are a key component to teaching scholarship, as they provide the context for situated learning and cognitive apprenticeship.

Because these traditions involve pursuing a line of inquiry *over time*, both faculty and students are continuously improving their skills and expertise. From the perspective of cognitive apprenticeship, the temporal and developmental aspects of our traditions of inquiry enable students to engage in progressively more challenging activities with mentors whom they can observe, consult, and challenge. As these processes and learning intersect, research teams are built, which benefits both faculty members and students.

Building the research team intersects with student projects, theses, and doctoral dissertations. Students are not expected to identify and pursue "original and independent" research; instead, research emanates from teams of mentors and learners with complementary knowledge and skills working together. Given our theory base of social learning, it makes sense that students learn research by participating in a process that reflects how quality applied research is done. Following this line of reasoning, student projects, theses, and dissertations are expected to emanate from one of the traditions of inquiry in the department.

At UIC, thesis and dissertation work are aimed at generating new knowledge or strengthening existing knowledge through replication or refinement of knowledge. Projects are aimed at applying knowledge to practice. Students choose a thesis or project depending on their career aims, and/or their desire to develop a research career through additional doctoral or post-doctoral level work. The identification of questions and methods for student work occurs through a number of avenues. Often students begin by working as research assistants or undertaking credit-generating activities that involve them at the ground level in a research project(s). Students have the opportunity to participate in informal interactions and to see the scholarship process unfold. They get an appreciation of what is being learned through the research and the inherent logic of the process. Identification of the student's thesis, dissertation, or project emanates from this tradition of inquiry and is developed within a community of scholars. In summary, the focus of student scholarship is generated in the same way that any new research questions or applications arise out of an ongoing program of research.

Moreover, when faculty members are advising students who are participating in their research tradition, they can effectively facilitate students' identification of research questions and methods. By advising students in areas of their own substantive and methodological expertise, the quality of the mentoring is enhanced. Moreover, because advisors are intellectually invested in the student's research or applied project, they are able to convey attitudes such as curiosity, patience, and tenacity, which drive quality scholarship.

The same kinds of benefits apply to student learning. Students who are further along in the process, and staff who are working on research projects, contribute to mentoring new students. Much of the tacit knowledge of doing research actually comes out of informal social interactions. Finally, because all members of a research team engage in ongoing discourse about the logistics, methods, questions, and findings of the research projects, students become fully immersed in a rich and dynamic learning environment.

The overall process we have just described enhances student learning and increases the quality of their research. It gives students the opportunity to make a meaningful contribution to a tradition of research. They see students ahead of them present research findings that stimulate their own questions, and help those behind them continue a line of investigation. A sense of belonging to an exciting research community is generated. Importantly, they become capable of contributing to cumulative knowledge development.

What should be obvious about this process is that students are not the only beneficiaries. Faculty's research traditions are greatly enhanced by having a pool of student collaborators. Because students often begin as research assistants and later conduct their research within a team, they become highly competent contributors given sustained involvement. Students who choose the project route help the team create applications relevant to practice and offer valuable products back to the research team and the community.

The following is one example of a tradition of research that has evolved through faculty and student work. This example also illustrates how two different lines of inquiry built upon each other. The two lines of inquiry are development of assessments for practice and understanding factors that affect vocational success. We began many years ago developing measures related to work success (Kielhofner, Lai, Olson, Haglund, Ekbadh & Hedlund, 1999; Velozo, Kielhofner, Gern, Lin, Azhar, Lai & Fisher, in press; Haglund, Karlsson, Kielhofner & Lai, 1999). At the same time we implemented and studied model work intervention programs. We documented these interventions in publications by faculty and students (Kielhofner, Braveman, Baron, Fisher, Hammel & Littleton, 1999; Mentrup, Neihaus & Kielhofner, 1999). With foundation funding, we conducted a study of one work program (Barrett, Beer & Kielhofner, 1999; Kielhofner & Barrett, 1997). Subsequently, we were contracted to conduct another pilot project, which applied and investigated our vocational approach with persons living with AIDS. Building on the experience, we obtained a three-year federal research grant to investigate the efficacy of this program.

This project is serving as a learning context for many students who are involved in data collection and analysis. Even as we are preparing to submit for a larger project, students are helping to collect and analyze pilot data to demonstrate need, search the literature to support arguments, and analyze findings from the ongoing study. Finally, the data collected are providing a foundation for several theses and dissertations.

Step #3: Making a Culture of Scholarly Collaboration Normative

The third step in operationalizing our approach to teaching scholarship was to create a culture where collaboration is valued and considered normative by faculty, graduate students, and practitioners. Interestingly, we faced, and continue to face, many challenges in trying to achieve this step.

Within academia, numerous barriers exist to creating a culture of collaboration, with the primary one being the myth of the independent researcher. The academy continues to hold the traditional ideal of the scholar as an independent researcher who makes a reputation for his/her original and unique work (Glassick, Huber & Maeroff, 1997). The mystique of this image still weighs on academic culture. It has influenced occupational therapy scholars and the extent to which their work is viewed as valuable by the profession. Such a notion of the independent scholar also widens the gap between academic researchers and practitioners and community members who question the validity of the "ivory tower" findings.

Additional barriers to developing a culture of scholarly collaboration are the realities that scholarship within academia is emotionally laden and competitive. The competitive component of scholarship also contributes to a phenomenon commonly referred to as the "silo" effect, that is, the tendency to limit interaction and scholarly discourse to individuals within one's discipline or narrow field of inquiry. Competition is a critical aspect of scholarship, from presentations to publications to grant writing. Both faculty and students are rewarded for their efforts through peer review, which is, by definition, competitive. While critical to the academic enterprise, competition and fear of having one's ideas "stolen" can prevent collaborative efforts from ever starting.

Another interesting barrier emanating largely from occupational therapy is the belief that integrating students into scholarly traditions, rather then sending them off to pursue their own research ideas, would stifle creativity or result in faculty members unfairly taking advantage of students to advance their own research agenda. These beliefs often persist despite the evidence to the contrary. Such evidence includes frustrated students who learn distaste for the research process, and the number of unpublished and unused works that emanate from the "independent and creative" model of student education and research. Our approach consistently yields graduate students who are finishing their graduate work in a timely manner, increasingly publishing and presenting their work in professional journals and public forums, and developing a commitment to research careers. This commitment is evidenced by the number of students who pursue advanced degrees, or who collaborate on ongoing research projects and grants.

Despite the barriers we have described, scholarly collaboration and teamwork are effectively fostered at UIC both within and outside the department. Key factors in achieving a collaborative environment are: (1) clear definition of roles and expectations, (2) maintaining clear ground rules for processes such as sharing and respecting ideas, credit, and co-publication, and (3) creating win-win situations in which all parties benefit.

Clear definition of roles and expectations. Collaboration occurs among and between the following groups: tenured and tenure-track faculty, clinical faculty, academic professionals (e.g., business manager), and graduate students. We have evolved a clear definition of the roles and responsibilities that go with each of these categories. For example, creating and sustaining research programs is a principle expectation of tenured and tenure-track faculty. Therefore, this group leads research activities within the department.

While research is not a central job responsibility of clinical faculty members, each one is involved in research in a different way (e.g., co-investigators, project coordinators, interventionists). This involvement stems from clinical faculty members' clinical expertise, research interests, and abilities to identify opportunities and negotiate job responsibilities and priorities (e.g., entry-level education, service). Currently, all clinical faculty are actively involved in research projects, publications, and presentations.

The academic professional staff play a significant role in the success of our scholarly efforts as they are the people who prepare grant budgets, negotiate procedures within the university, handle and coordinate the logistics of getting a grant out on time, and manage a grant once it is obtained.

Clinical staff often serve as data collectors and/or service providers in intervention studies. While clinical staff are not expected to generate or lead research, they actively participate in identifying or shaping research questions. In some of our traditions of inquiry such as developing assessments, the clinical staff are important resources for helping to shape and test the practicality and feasibility of the tools we develop.

Through their projects and thesis/dissertation work, students actively contribute to the scholarship. By working on an established line of research, students can replicate or expand upon findings and thus contribute to the knowledge base. In addition, many students take on roles as research assistantships, working as research coordinators, data collectors, data entry specialists, and data analysts.

Finally, members of the community play critical roles in our community of scholarship. Staff, administrators, and consumers from many community groups and organizations actively create and shape our scholarship, offering insider perspectives to everyday issues experienced in the urban community. We negotiate with them to validate their roles via inclusion in research and training grants, participant and agency reimbursement for involvement in research activities, and teaching appointments and honoraria.

Maintaining clear ground rules. With so many people contributing toward research we have found it useful to develop clear ground rules for how information is shared, what things can be copied or used by other researchers, and how credit is attributed in such things as grant investigator status and publication. We have a policy that governs student-faculty and multiple-author publications that provides co-publication guidelines that have evolved over time. This policy serves to introduce students to the concept of authorship and to the principles that guide decisions about it. It also outlines procedures for deciding authorship.

A second example of how we have handled sharing information and academic credit is the detailed guidelines we developed to facilitate collaboration and free sharing of information through our Center of Outcomes Research and Education, which involves a community of seventeen fellows from universities in the United States, Canada, and Sweden, and a network of graduate students working with them. We routinely share scholarly products, such as drafts of grant proposals or grant reviews, so we can critically analyze them as a group and offer feedback. Consequently, we developed by consensus the following ground rules:

1. When anyone provides written materials to the group as part of sharing ideas, he/she should specify any limitations on its use/copying/distribution. This information should be stated on the information shared.
2. When someone wishes to limit handouts to a discussion context, he/she may distribute them during the seminar and then take them back after the presentation.
3. It is important that we respect each other's work and, in particular, respect ownership of original ideas. Whenever it is not clear, the expected ground rule is to consult with the original author in regard to citing, sharing, or building upon any of his/her work.

By developing careful ground rules for how members will access, use, and limit distribution of such materials, we have been able to achieve a sense of safety and freedom in how we share information.

Creating win-win situations. Many of the same factors that create competition in scholarship can also create a feeling that scholarship is a zero-sum game. For example, only so many grant dollars will be distributed to competing scholars. However, there are many other aspects of research that involve mutual benefit. When scholars share resources, stimulate and critique each other, and build from each other's learning and success, everyone benefits. This article is a good example. No single one of us had the resources to write this article alone. However, we agreed that we wanted to share the information it contains. We divided up tasks, shared responsibilities for writing, discussed how we wanted to structure it, and critiqued each other's contributions. By pooling our collective resources, we were able to produce something that allowed each contributor to benefit.

When members of a community come to expect that working together will yield mutual benefits, collaboration becomes more frequent, enjoyable, and productive. The following is another example of how win-win situations are created that extend beyond faculty members to students and community members. Two faculty members, one on tenure track and one on clinical track, began collaborating on a grant to explore the occupational strategies utilized by older adults to stay in the home and community. They partnered with the local

Department on Aging and Senior Center to implement a life history group to explore these strategies, while helping older adults share their own stories. Several students became involved in different roles such as facilitating the group, helping seniors record their narratives, and designing a Web site to share these stories. The older adults in the project took on roles as mentors to faculty and students, teaching them about aging in the urban context and ensuring that the research reflected their experience.

This initial project led to several pilot studies on life role development and resource management among older adults who experienced significant disability events. These pilot studies supported a successful National Institute on Aging grant to study a group of older adults returning home after a stroke. This grant involves collaboration with a senior professor from another department who offers longitudinal research expertise to the project, and who has since collaborated on several other research studies in the department.

As shown in this example, we have sought to create win-win relationships with others in our college and university and with other community collaborators and organizations. Outcomes of these collaborations have included grants, publications, presentations, and educational activities that are integrated across our curriculum.

Step #4: Creating Research, Teaching, and Service Synergies

Faculty and students have multiple responsibilities and demands on their time. As a result, productivity and learning can be put at risk if scholarly efforts are not synergistic and instead move in competing directions. Synergistic efforts are those which serve multiple and complementary purposes. Examples of such efforts include offering continuing education courses that provide the opportunity to develop research ideas or disseminate findings, and integrating participation in a research project (e.g., collecting or analyzing data) as part of a course requirement.

Often synergies are created on a larger scale when we develop relationships that serve more than a single purpose. Sometimes relationships that begin with faculty research later provide opportunities for student projects or theses. On other occasions what began as a relationship focused on teaching and service later opened avenues for research. For example, a tradition of inquiry that focused on program evaluation (Beer & Helfrich, 1996) placed research faculty in the community in settings where occupational therapy did not exist. Through involvement with these various community agencies, faculty identified potential opportunities for education. Developing student placements there brought valuable resources to the agency. The enhanced relationship between the department and the agency served as a foundation for opportunities to do research.

We have also actively involved community members as guest lecturers and developed stimulating case materials for our curriculum. The richness of these settings allows students to take advantage of the cognitive apprenticeships as they complete useful and interesting projects, such as case study modules and targeted program development for specific populations alongside a faculty member conducting research.

Another approach to synergizing efforts at UIC can be illustrated through the outcomes of student theses and projects. As part of the cognitive apprenticeship approach, students enter a faculty member's research tradition. This allows both research and clinical faculty to further their efforts through effective mentoring of student advisees and research assistants. In the previous example, a clinical faculty member might assign a student to complete a project to develop a case study for a course they are teaching, or create a module for the class related to a specific topic. Research faculty work with theses students to identify a component of their research to complete as thesis and work with project students to identify aspects of application that will contribute to developing practice. These efforts guide students in how to apply research findings to practice.

As faculty we have slowly developed the ability to creatively envision the next steps in our research and what we need to do to get there. By identifying steps such as pilot study data collection and products such as papers or analysis needed for future grant submissions, we can provide students with an array of projects or thesis topics from which to choose. When students are working on projects related to our work, the effort we expend in advising becomes both an investment in the student and in our future as academicians. This model provides students with hands-on experience contributing to the progression of a research tradition.

The final step to synergizing our efforts is to create apprenticeship opportunities for students through the process of dissemination. An example of this process occurred with a tenure track faculty member working in the area of domestic violence. All of her advisees completed projects or theses related to domestic abuse. In addition, students in her graduate seminars completed papers related to the same topic. By running a writing group focused on the issue of domestic violence that was composed of students, recent graduates and collaborating faculty, seven papers comprising a special issue of *Occupational Therapy in Mental Health* were completed (Helfrich, in press). The papers ranged from theoretical pieces authored by the faculty member to case illustrations and applications of tools developed by her students (Helfrich & Aviles, in press; Helfrich, Lafata, MacDonald, Aviles & Collins, in press; Johnston, Adams & Helfrich, in press; Lafata & Helfrich, in press; MacDonald & Helfrich, in press; Nave, Helfrich & Aviles, in press; Walens, Helfrich, Aviles & Horita, in press). The outcome of these efforts was highly productive for the faculty member while developing a foundation of publications on which to build further research. This type of dissemination provides scholarship to our research, service, and teaching efforts while contributing to our productivity. In addition, it provides a situated learning opportunity for our students to learn writing skills as well as the skills needed to participate in a dynamic and critical scholarly interchange with their peers and faculty.

Step #5: Creating Vehicles for Idea Development and Constructive Commentary

Scholarly careers can seem masochistic to an outsider. From the time of having to *defend* a thesis or dissertation plan and product to the ritual of peer review of manuscripts and grant proposals with all their attendant criticism, rejection, and refusal, faculty and students cannot be blamed for "running for cover." Nonetheless, debate and criticism are fundamental processes whereby scholarship is kept honest. If these processes can be done within a supportive community of practice and be seen as facilitating the scholar and the methods of scholarship, they can be turned into something positive and productive. Moreover, this kind of context is necessary for students who are novices to the research process to feel comfortable about learning. Creating the right atmosphere for developing scholarship in general results in an optimal learning environment.

To this end, we have implemented multiple vehicles for sharing and critiquing our scholarship with fellow faculty, students, practitioners, and community members. A weekly symposium is held to highlight ideas for research and seek feedback, to present applied case studies linking research to practice, to share emerging results from a study or grant in progress, or to disseminate results of completed research. Students, faculty, and practitioners who present hone their ability to articulate their scholarship, and to respond to critiques. All participate in the discussions and, over time, increase their comfort with offering and receiving informed critiques of the work presented. Students receive credit for attending these and other colloquiums throughout the university every semester, thus validating the importance of this situated learning activity.

We also invite scholars from outside the department or university to present work that is related to our scholarship, and to discuss how research traditions from other disciplines can be applied. These activities help us to mitigate the "silo effect" so common in occupational therapy, and open the potential for collaborating on interdisciplinary research. They also increase our awareness of other research traditions so we are not "recreating the wheel" but instead, are building upon, and acknowledging, existing scholarship.

In addition to attendance and participation in the colloquium series, students are expected to demonstrate their articulation and critical analysis skills by presenting the outcomes of their work in multiple forums. Since students who do these presentations will have already seen other students, faculty, and others do such presentations and receive feedback, they are much more comfortable and informed about the process. Rather than viewing these as difficult rites of passage, students tend to view them as opportunities to develop professional presentation skills and share their work with a community of interested colleagues.

Another important vehicle that we have developed to encourage and enhance idea development within the department is writing groups, each of which focuses on a particular content or methodology area. Recently, we have invited scholars from other disciplines to facilitate writing groups aimed at increasing peer-reviewed publication submissions. These groups provide opportunities for faculty and students to further hone and critique writing skills that are critical for disseminating knowledge. In addition, these groups sustain opportunities for ongoing scholarly development. This development is necessary to ensure that we remain on the cutting edge methodologically, in practice, and in the way we design education for our students.

CONCLUSION

This article described an approach to educating new scholars that emphasizes creation of a cumulative body of knowledge with relevance to practice. Our approach is based on social learning theory and is actively applied through situated learning and cognitive apprenticeship strategies. The foundation of the approach is a dynamic scholarly community of learning. We identified five key steps to creating such a community.

This approach enhances both faculty productivity and student learning. It has enabled faculty members to develop substantive and methodological expertise and resources over time, to increase their abilities to compete for grant funding, and to engage in research that is recognized by interdisciplinary peers. From a broader perspective, the application of the approach has enabled the faculty to contribute to the cumulative knowledge of the profession of occupational therapy. By having faculty and students work together to build a tradition of inquiry, there is growing empirical support for occupational therapy, both theoretically and practically. These group efforts, and the synergies and collaborations we actively seek with our interdisciplinary colleagues and community partners, provide the opportunity to develop and enhance the ideas and concepts that will take occupational therapy into this millennium.

REFERENCES

Abreu, B.C., Peloquin, S.M., & Ottenbacher, K. (1998). Competence in scientific inquiry and research. *The American Journal of Occupational Therapy, 52* (9), 751-759.

Anderson, J.R., Reder, L.M., & Simon, H.A. (1996). Situated learning and education. *Educational Researcher, 24* (4), 5-11.

Barrett, L., Beer, D., & Kielhofner, G. (1999). The importance of volitional narrative in treatment: An ethnographic case study in a work program. *Work: A Journal of Prevention, Assessment & Rehabilitation, 12*, 79-92.

Beer, D.W., & Helfrich, C.A. (1996). *Evaluation of Ridgeland Enhanced Head Start program for transitional housing residents.* Final Report, U.S. Department of Health and Human Services.

Berryman, S.E. (1990). *Designing effective learning environments: Cognitive apprenticeship models.* New York, NY: Institute on Education and the Economy.

Brown, A.L. (1994). The advancement of learning. *Educational Researcher, 23* (8), 4-12.

Brown, J.S., Collins, A., & Duguid, P. (1989). Situated cognition and the culture of learning. *Educational Researcher, 18*(1), 32-41.

Case-Smith, J. (1999). Developing a research career: Advice from occupational therapy researchers. *American Journal of Occupational Therapy, 53*, 44-50.

Christiansen, C. (1981). Toward revolution of crisis: Research requisites in occupational therapy. *The Occupational Therapy Journal of Research, 1*, 115-124.

Christiansen, C. (1990). The perils of plurality. *The Occupational Therapy Journal of Research, 10*, 259-265.

Collins, A. (1991). Cognitive apprenticeship and instructional technology. In L. Idol & B.F. Jones (Eds.), *Educational values and cognitive instruction: Implications for reform.* Hillsdale, NJ: Lawrence Erlbaum Associates.

Collins, A., Brown, J.S., & Newman, S. (1989). Cognitive apprenticeship: Teaching the craft of reading, writing, and mathematics. In L.B. Resnick (Ed.), *Knowing, learning and instruction: Essays in honor of Robert Glaser.* Hillsdale, NJ: Lawrence Erlbaum Associates.

Dunn, W., Brown, C., & McGuigan, A. (1994). The ecology of human performance: A framework for considering the effect of context. *The American Journal of Occupational Therapy, 48* (7), 595-607.

Glassick, C.E., Huber, M.T., & Maeroff, G.I. (1997). Scholarship assessed: Evaluation of the professoriate. San Francisco: Jossey-Bass.

Haglund, L., Karlsson, G., Kielhofner, G., & Lai, J.S. (1997). Validity of the Swedish version of the Worker Role Interview. *Scandinavian Journal of Occupational Therapy, 4*, 23-29.

Hammel, J. (2000). Linking ICIDH-2 and OT theory to everyday practice. *Annual Illinois OT Assocation Conference*, Galena, IL, Oct. 31, 2000.

Helfrich, C.A. (Ed.) (2001). *Occupational Therapy in Mental Health, Volume 16* (3/4).

Helfrich, C.A., & Aviles, A. (2001). Occupational therapy's role with victims of domestic violence: Assessment and intervention. *Occupational Therapy in Mental Health, 16* (3/4).

Helfrich, C.A., Lafata, M.J., MacDonald, A.L., Aviles, A., & Collins, L. (2001). Domestic abuse across the lifespan: The role of occupational therapy. *Occupational Therapy in Mental Health, 16* (3/4).

Johnston, J.L., Adams, R., & Helfrich, C.A. (2001). Knowledge and attitudes of occupational therapy practitioners regarding wife abuse. *Occupational Therapy in Mental Health, 16* (3/4).

Kemper, T. D. (2000). Toward Sociology as a Science. *Chronicle of Higher Education. The Chronicle Review.* August 11.

Kennedy, D. (1997). *Academic duty.* Cambridge, MA: Harvard University Press.

Kielhofner, G. (2000). *A scholarship of practice: How knowledge development can best serve practice in the new millennium.* Keynote Address. British Occupational Therapy Annual Conference, Keele, England, July 18, 2000.

Kielhofner, G. (1997). *Conceptual foundations of occupational therapy* (2nd Ed.). Philadelphia: F.A. Davis.

Kielhofner, G. (1995). *A model of human occupation: Theory and application* (2nd Ed.). Baltimore: Williams & Wilkins.

Kielhofner, G., & Barrett, L. (1997). Meaning and misunderstanding in occupational forms: A study of therapeutic goal setting. *The American Journal of Occupational Therapy, 52,* 345-353.

Kielhofner, G., Braveman, B., Baron, K., Fisher, G., Hammel, J., & Littleton, M. (1999). The model of human occupation: Understanding the worker who is injured or disabled. *Work, 12,* 3-12.

Kielhofner, G., Lai, J.S., Olson, L., Haglund, L., Ekbadh, E., & Hedlund, M. (1999). Psychometric properties of the work environment impact scale: A cross-cultural study. *Work, 12,* 71-78.

Kirschner, D., & Whitson, J. (Eds). (1997). *Situated cognition: Social, semiotic, and psychological perspectives.* Mahwah, NJ: Lawrence Erlbaum Associates.

Lafata, M.J., & Helfrich, C.A. (2001). The occupational therapy elder abuse checklist. *Occupational Therapy in Mental Health, 16* (3/4).

Lave, J. (1988). *Cognition in practice.* New York, NY: Cambridge Press.

Lave, J. (1997). The culture of acquisition and the practice of understanding. In D. Kirschner & J. Whitson (Eds.), *Situated cognition: Social, semiotic, and psychological perspectives,* 17-35. Mahwah, NJ: Lawrence Erlbaum Associates.

Lave, J., & Wenger, E. (1991). *Situated learning.* New York, NY: Cambridge Press.

Law, M., Cooper, B., Strong, S., Stewart, D., Rigby, P., & Letts, L. (1996). The person-environment-occupation model: A transactive approach to occupational performance. *The Canadian Journal of Occupational Therapy, 63* (1), 9-23.

Lieberman, A. (1993). The meaning of scholarly activity and the building of community. *Equity & Choice, 10* (1), 4-10.

MacDonald, S.L., & Helfrich, C.A. (2001). Shaken baby syndrome: Assessing and treatment in occupational therapy. *Occupational Therapy in Mental Health, 16* (3/4).

Mentrup, C., Neihaus, A., & Kielhofner, G. (1999). Applying the model of human occupation in work-focused rehabilitation: A case illustration. *Work, 12,* 61-70.

Nave, J., Helfrich, C.A., & Aviles, A. (2001). Child witness domestic violence: A case study using the OT PAL. *Occupational Therapy in Mental Health, 16* (3/4).

Nelson, D. (1988). Occupation: Form and performance. *American Journal of Occupational Therapy, 42* (10): 633-641.

Schkade, J.K., & Schultz, S. (1992). Occupational adaptation: Toward a holistic approach for contemporary practice, part 1. *The American Journal of Occupational Therapy, 46,* 829-837.

Schultz, S., & Schkade, J.K. (1992). Occupational adaptation: Toward a holistic approach for contemporary practice, part 2. *The American Journal of Occupational Therapy, 46,* 917-925.

Stein, D. (1998). *Situated learning in adult education.* ERIC Digest No. 195, 1-6.

Townsend, E. (Ed.). (1997). *Enabling occupation: An occupational therapy perspective.* Ottawa, ON: CAOT/ACE Publications.

UIC Department of Occupational Therapy. (2000). A scholarship of practice. Available on the world wide web at: http://www.uic.edu/ahp/OT/researcha.htm

Velozo, C., Kielhofner, G., Gern, A., Lin, F-L, Azhar, F., Lai, J-S, & Fisher, G. (1999). Worker Role Interview: Validation of a psychosocial work-related measure. *Journal of Occupational Rehabilitation, 9,* 153-168.

Vygotsky, L.S. (1978). *Mind in society: The development of higher psychological processes.* Cambridge, MA: Harvard University Press.

Walens, D., Helfrich, C. A., Aviles, A., & Horita, L. (2001). Assessing needs and developing interventions with new populations: A community process of collaboration. *Occupational Therapy in Mental Health, 16* (3/4).

Willemsen, E.W., & Gainen, J. (1995). Reenvisioning statistics: A cognitive apprenticeship approach. *New Directions for Teaching and Learning, 61,* 99-108.

Wilson, A. (1993). The promise of situated cognition. In: S.B. Merriam (Ed.), *An update on adult learning theory,* 71-79. San Francisco, CA: Jossey-Bass.

Young, M.F. (1993). Instructional design for situated learning. *Educational Technology Research and Development, 41* (1), 43-58.

Zemke, R., & Clark, F. (1996). *Occupational Science: The evolving discipline.* Philadelphia, PA: F.A. Davis.

Qualitative Evaluation
of a Management Course Project:
Creating New Job Possibilities
for Occupational Therapy

Patricia L. Schaber, MA, OTR/L

SUMMARY. A qualitative analysis of a ten-step management course project in occupational therapy education demonstrates the students changed perception of future job possibilities. The assignment, designed using a student-centered approach, bridges individual skills and interests with the creation of an occupational therapy position in an emerging market. The thematic analysis indicated the outcomes of the assignment were: a changed perception in the importance of a *good fit* between practitioner skills and the agency or program needs, added *confidence* in the students' skills based on a review of the two years of academic education, and a positive, anticipated *transition* of the academic knowledge base into real world experience. Student presentations served to measure the ability to articulate the services of occupational therapy within arenas unfamiliar to the profession. *[Article copies available for a fee from The Haworth Document Delivery Service: 1-800-HAWORTH. E-mail address: <getinfo@haworthpressinc.com> Website: <http://www.HaworthPress.com> © 2001 by The Haworth Press, Inc. All rights reserved.]*

Patricia L. Schaber is Instructor, Program in Occupational Therapy, University of Minnesota, MMC 388, Minneapolis, MN 55455 (E-mail: schab002@tc.umn.edu).

[Haworth co-indexing entry note]: "Qualitative Evaluation of a Management Course Project: Creating New Job Possibilities for Occupational Therapy." Schaber, Patricia L. Co-published simultaneously in *Occupational Therapy in Health Care* (The Haworth Press, Inc.) Vol. 15, No. 1/2, 2001, pp. 177-192; and: *Education for Occupational Therapy in Health Care: Strategies for the New Millennium* (eds: Patricia Crist, and Marjorie Scaffa) The Haworth Press, Inc., 2001, pp. 177-192. Single or multiple copies of this article are available for a fee from The Haworth Document Delivery Service [1-800-HAWORTH, 9:00 a.m. - 5:00 p.m. (EST). E-mail address: getinfo@haworthpressinc.com].

KEYWORDS. Management course project, emerging markets, management education

The occupational therapy profession has experienced growing pains in the last decade, not unlike other decades (Jacobs, 2000; Christiansen, 1975). Medicare's Prospective Payment System of 1998, Individuals With Disabilities Education Act of 1997, State Medicaid guidelines, and changes in service coverage of health maintenance organizations (HMOs) have all made an impact on how occupational therapists practice (American Occupational Therapy Association [AOTA], 1996; Foto, 1998; AOTA, 1999). An occupational therapy student graduating today is faced with an oversupply of professionals in the job market and less demand in traditionally served areas (Steib, 1999). This scenario has altered the demands on the entry level graduate and created a need for development of competencies in new arenas (Loukas, 2000). What new graduates need today is confidence in their skills to serve populations outside of the traditional medical model, the ability to translate the skills learned in an academic program to a job of their own design, and competence in articulating the skills of an occupational therapy practitioner to community-based agencies. This article will describe a community-based management project designed to incorporate the development of these competencies in a manner that challenges the students at their level during the last semester of the academic portion of the curriculum.

The management course project is uniquely designed to tap into the student-centered interests and skills that each student brings to the profession. A creativity exercise, "clustering," initiates the project to guide students to think in terms of creating a job to fit their skills and interests versus the student fitting an established position. Each student is then guided to identify an emerging market for occupational therapy (OT) services that does not presently employ an OT practitioner. The challenge for the students as they progress through the 10-step process lies in their attempt to articulate the "edge" they bring to the position they have created and identify the skills that were developed within the OT curriculum that serve it. The final product, a 15-minute multimedia presentation, serves as a culmination of the academic portion of the program as students pull together the threads of OT education into creative, exciting possibilities of what the future may hold. The assignment is intended to alter student perceptions and launch the student into a sea of possibilities rather than a quagmire of limitations.

The objectives of the project are threefold:

1. To expand the students' perceptions that the jobs of OT can be created or adapted to their unique abilities and passions as they redefine their skills outside of a medical or institutional model.
2. To instill a sense of confidence in the students that they can translate their two years of academic training into a job opportunity in the real-world practice of the profession.
3. To culminate the program with the ability to articulate the services of the profession within arenas unfamiliar with OT in that setting.

The method of analysis selected for evaluating the first two objectives, which measured changes in students perception, was a qualitative approach (Miles & Huberman, 1988). Data included text material obtained using open-ended questions in a short essay format. The third objective was measured by rating the students' 15-minute presentations of the job positions created for an emerging market. This rating coded the ability of the student to articulate OT services and the community center's receptivity to the idea of incorporating OT services within their agency. As a standard curriculum evaluation method, a focus group of the class project was conducted to stimulate suggestions regarding how the assignment could be improved for future students.

Other management competencies embedded within the assignment include creating a job description, identifying skill attainment, performing a community-based needs assessment, interviewing, and presenting.

HISTORY OF THE MANAGEMENT PROJECT

Project assignments in the course, *Management of Occupational Therapy Services,* have reflected the state of the profession and the OT skills demanded of that era. In the more distant past, the 1980s, the management course project consisted of creating a hypothetical OT clinic where application of information in topic areas such as staffing, cost accounting, budgeting, inventory, and supervision were the focus (course syllabi archives). The project reflected the needs of the time, for OT practitioners to graduate with the skills to set up their own clinics, as occupational therapy branched into rural areas and expanded diversification in health-care facilities.

After clinical sites saturated the industry, the need arose for OT practitioners to think beyond the traditional clinical intervention services to the creation of "innovative" programs to serve clients in the existing health-care facilities that were underserved. The purpose of the management project during this period, the 1990s, was to create an innovative program in an OT setting that went beyond the scope of services presently offered, yet remained within the context of the traditional OT environment. The outcome was demonstration of skills in needs assessment and program development. Once more, the project used the creation of a hypothetical program format that could creatively serve the existing clientele in a new way. The problem with this assignment was that the student required additional coaching to come up with a program idea that was innovative due to the limited amount of clinical exposure the students had to draw upon for new ideas.

The challenge facing academic educators today, bridging the gap between the knowledge base of the curriculum and professional competencies in the field, is in making the experiences relevant to the challenges facing prospective graduates. In the present curricular model, students gain a solid base of experience through fieldwork in the more traditional settings and optional fieldwork experiences and, with the management project, have the added ability to translate the knowledge and skills into a new environment. The project is intended to expand the possibilities within the emerging markets of occupational therapy.

THE ASSIGNMENT

This is a multi-step assignment that spans the entire semester, from idea formulation in the first week through the project presentations scheduled in the last three weeks. It is the major project for the course (30% of the grade), which includes other assignments: an ethical reflection paper (10%), a resume and cover letter (10%), a unit 1 exam (25%), and unit 2 exam (25%). Each step of the project is introduced within the course topic material and some of the steps are completed within class time. Ongoing class discussion of student progress is encouraged and a timeline is given to the students to stay on track for different steps of the project.

Step 1. The student participates in an in-class clustering exercise (Boyd, 1995). The purpose is to draw on the areas of strength and interest within each student. It begins with a brief meditation followed by a free association of words relating to a "career." The exercise is designed to release individual creativity through self-reflection. (See Figure 1.)

Step 2. The student identifies an agency or community group where this interest can be realized. It may be an agency the student is familiar with, but oftentimes it requires some investigation. The only stipulation is that the agency must provide a service where the skills of an occupational therapist would benefit the clients or personnel.

FIGURE 1. Clustering Technique

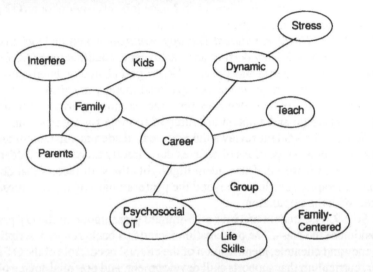

Clustering technique–Use free association to create a visual pathway of words that have meaning to the topical word that serves as a starting point. Then create a paragraph combining words to make goals for yourself.

I want a **career** that can accommodate having a **family** and **kids** and room for my **parents** but I don't want them to **interfere**. I like **psychosocial OT** especially when it is working with **groups** on **life skills** and I appreciate the **family centered** approach. I want a job that's **dynamic**, even though that comes with more **stress**. Maybe I'd like to **teach** someday or incorporate teaching into my career.

Step 3. The student receives approval of the idea from the instructor of the course. This individual meeting serves as an opportunity for the students to begin to articulate their vision of occupational therapy service with the identified population.

Step 4. The student investigates the agency/community program, gathering information on the vision, mission or purpose, organizational structure, and existing programs. The investigation identifies the population served, the client needs, the sources of funding for the existing programs, and situates the agency within the services provided by the greater community. The needs assessment is application of a process the students theoretically learned in a *Community Resources* course. The student identifies a key informant and schedules an interview with that person.

Step 5. The student interviews the key informant. The interview includes an explanation of the assignment, articulation of occupational therapy services, investigation of the needs of the clients, and a response from the key informant as to how that individual could visualize occupational therapy services utilized within the agency.

Step 6. The student develops a 1 to 2 page job description for an OT practitioner position within the agency or community group. It incorporates the format presented in *The Occupational Therapy Manager* which includes major function, scope of role, key performance areas, and qualifications (AOTA, 1996). The job title may be expanded, i.e., OTR/Program Director, but the job prerequisite includes skills requiring an occupational therapy practitioner.

Step 7. The student identifies both the existing source of funding of the agency/program and a potential source of funding for the position.

Step 8. The student reviews the two-year academic curriculum and identifies the courses or portions of courses that directly serve the skill development for the job identified. The student highlights the skill factors that an occupational therapist contributes beyond the professional staffing mix presently utilized with the population.

Step 9. The student prepares a 15-minute presentation of the OT practitioner position to the class. The presentation includes a background description of the agency and clientele, identification of the clients' needs, role of the OT practitioner, curriculum that supports skill development, and potential source of funding for the position. The audience is future employers, and the presentation package is intended to be usable in a future job search. The presentation may be with computer projection, overheads, or handout materials. For each presentation, a fellow student presents a brief five-minute response to the project idea, commenting on feasibility and identifying areas needing further clarification.

Step 10. The student submits a written report (6 to 10 pages) with the following information:

- Organizational evaluation–2 to 3 pages (vision, mission, or brochures can be included in the addendum)
- Analysis of program–1 to 2 pages
- Development of job description–1 to 2 pages
- Synthesizing the OT curricular knowledge base with the new position–2 to 3 pages. (See Table 1.)

The paper is graded using the following criteria:

1. Creativity–10 points (Demonstration of clustering technique or other method to explore your career interests that point you to a particular set-

ting, population, or type of work. The idea is innovative, feasible, interesting.)

2. Vision, mission, and organizational structure–20 points (Vision and mission statement included along with future directions or strategic plan. Organizational structure and key roles of those administering the agency are summarized.)
3. Program description–10 points (Thorough identification of the program(s) and the populations served by the agency. Skills developed in *Community Resources* used effectively in assessing the agency and the needs of the clients.)
4. Job description–20 points (Job description accurately reflects the position and skills identified, demonstrating consistency with title, level of responsibility, and performance tasks. Student has a clear idea of what the job would entail.)
5. Application of curriculum to emerging market–20 points (Knowledge and skills identified from the curriculum in the occupational therapy program support the tasks identified in the job description. Unique contribution of OT to the position identified.)
6. Class presentation–20 points (Skills developed in the *Adult Education* course used effectively in the creation of a formal 15-minute presentation.)

EVALUATION METHOD

Questionnaire

The method of evaluation used to measure objective 1 (a personalized redefinition of skills in a nontraditional environment) and objective 2 (a sense of

TABLE 1. The Management Project Summarized

Ten Step Management Project
Step 1. Clustering: self-reflection to discover area of interest
Step 2. Choose agency, center, or program
Step 3. Approval of project idea from the instructor
Step 4. Investigation of the agency: vision, mission, and programs
Step 5. Interview key informant on site
Step 6. Create OT practitioner job description
Step 7. Identify funding source for position
Step 8. Review academic curriculum for sources of skill development
Step 9. Create a 15-minute presentation
Step 10. Write report

confidence and opportunity) is a descriptive approach using textual analysis of a written response to an open-ended questionnaire (Miles & Huberman, 1997). From the questionnaires, pattern codes were identified, grouping words with similar meaning to create thematic categorical areas. Sentences or phrases supporting the theme were grouped in a table. Participation in the written questionnaire was optional.

In the questionnaire, students were asked to respond to the following questions:

1. Identify any portion of the management project that you found valuable. Explain why it was valuable. Probes listing the steps of the project were included to encourage them to think of the entire assignment.
2. What were the unanticipated outcomes of the assignment? What did participation in this assignment do for you?

Evaluating Presentations

Objective 3 (competence in articulating the skills of an occupational therapist in a new setting) was evaluated by rating how well the student could articulate the role of OT in their presentations in class, the paired student response, and by gauging the agency's response to the student, as subjectively reported by the student interviewer. It was recorded if the agency was favorable or reluctant to view OT as a potential service that could serve a need within the facility.

Focus Group

Finally, a focus group of the entire class was conducted to stimulate suggestions regarding what worked and what did not, how the assignment could be improved for future students, and overall impressions of the experience. This was an instructor-facilitated session with recorded field notes from the discussion. Because not all students completed the written questionnaire, this was an opportunity to validate the written responses of the group that responded and to include verbal responses from other students who may not have had the same impression of the assignment.

RESULTS

Questionnaire

The thematic categories that emerged from a qualitative analysis of the written text support that the objectives anticipated by the assignment were successfully met. The class was made up of 23 students, and 14 responded to the written questionnaire. Of the 14 respondents, the following thematic categories emerged.

A Good Fit

The first theme generated was that the job created by the student was *a good fit*. It appears that personalizing the process by starting with an exploration of the unique interests and strengths of the student served as a strong motivator in the process (see Table 2). One student referred to the process as "discovering my own emerging market." Comments were made that the student infrequently has the freedom within the curriculum to select a project so individualized. Rather than encountering student complaints about the "burden" of finding a source to interview, the students seemed excited when the interview date was approaching. One student volunteered for a weekend at the local homeless shelter assisting the staff, visiting with the clients, and playing cards. He then interviewed a social service staff person after that experience. He commented:

> This assignment provided me with an opportunity (excuse) to learn more about the homeless–something I have been meaning to do but lacked the motivation.

The project appeared to open their vision of job possibilities beyond the medical model and school settings. Another student referred to it as "thinking outside of the box." One student pointed out that educators limit the vision of job possibilities by their selection of in-class examples:

> I feel that we focused on mainstream or common OT settings in most class examples, but through the individual research we did in management class it is apparent that there are many nontraditional settings that OTs can tap into.

The students were initially given the opportunity to pair up with another student who shared a similar interest area. None of the students took this option, and each of the projects was quite individualized.

When the students began to explore the various agencies or programs, their initial reaction was a hesitation toward the feasibility of an OT in this setting. Although they could see a connection with OT skills and the population served, how this could be realized in a job in the agency was a more distant leap.

TABLE 2. The Center/Agency Name and the Title of the OT Practitioner Position in the Job Description

Center/Agency	Job Title/OT Practitioner
Minnesota Diversified Industries (adult opportunity workshop)	Ergonomic Consultant
Region 9–AOA (county aging services)	Home Safety Consultant
YMCA Fitness Center	Senior Program Coordinator
Sylvan Learning Centers	Director of Special Services
Center for Independent Living	Marketing Specialist
Eau Claire Academy (adolescent treatment)	Skills Trainer
Natural Body Healing & Botanical Center	OT Consultant and Therapist
St. Paul Center for Handicapped Accessibility	Home and Environmental Coordinator
Grandparents as Parents Program	Human Services Coordinator
Lifetime Fitness	Stress Management Consultant
Catholic Charities (homeless drop-in center)	Activity Coordinator
Spa Montage	Life Skills Trainer
Chrysalis Women's Center (abuse survivors)	Counselor/OTR
In Touch Rehab & Chiropractic	Myofascial Release Therapist
Cancer Rehab Clinic—Outpatient Tx	OTR & Lymphedema Specialist
Mpls Crisis Nursery (temporary shelter)	Program Director
Pillsbury Company	Employee Assistance Consultant
Chrestomathy Center (adult DD day Tx)	Program Coordinator
Fetal Alcohol Syndrome Diagnostic Center	OTR Evaluator
Center for Spirituality and Healing	Educational Coordinator
Bridgehouse (adolescent residential treatment)	Unit Director
GRECC Center (sheltered workshop for clients with Alzheimer's disease)	Program Coordinator
Industrial OT	Ergonomics & ADA Consultant

I think the most valuable part of the assignment was finding where we would fit in an organization and developing a job description to meet the organization's needs. Many of us can see that OT belongs in many new settings, but taking it a step further to see exactly how we can meet their needs, proved challenging and valuable.

The written comments indicate that the in-class student presentations were the strongest vehicle promoting opportunities in emerging markets. The presentations also highlighted how the job can be tailored to the unique skills and personalities of the presenters. The students often commented on how they could visualize the student presenter performing in that position. They gained a new sense of respect for the diversity of their student group.

> Prior to this assignment, I thought about trying to find a job that fits my interests and skills. Now, I think about creating the job that allows me to follow my passions, use my skills and develop my career in the direction I choose.

> When listening to the presentations, I really realized how very diverse OT is and how OT is a perfect fit in many settings.

What emerged was a changed perception in how the agency could adapt to or support their skills rather than anticipating that they would conform to an established job. Finding a "good fit" became more important.

> This [the assignment] will allow us to determine where our expertise fits within the agency and whether it is a good match for us.

> . . . focusing on the program where OT can fill an identified need and present the strengths that OT can bring. There were many options to choose–finding the right or appropriate fit was the challenge.

Confidence and Opportunity

Bridging the link between the cognitive side of professional training and the application side has generally created anxiety among students leaving the academic institution. The second theme that emerged was *instilling confidence* in the student that the skills they acquired can serve a population within and outside of the traditional medical model.

> The assignment gave me some confidence to promote OT. I want to work in an emerging market so I thought the assignment was *great* practice.

> Overall, I was very excited about the assignment and especially the confidence I saw in myself and my classmates in terms of the future of our profession.

The students pointed out that their source of confidence came from the portion of the assignment requiring that they review the academic portion of the curriculum relative to skill development. The courses most frequently identified were courses that the students had previously reported to have less value or less applicability to OT, such as Group Dynamics, Community Resources, Management, and Adult Education.

> Simply analyzing the courses which I have taken the past two years increased my self-confidence. I am able to see the skills and abilities I have

acquired and I am now much more secure as to what I have to offer as an occupational therapist.

Going through classes for the past two years made me realize how much I learned and boosted my confidence in preparation for fieldwork.

The hope was that the experience would empower students to launch into fieldwork on an optimistic note and to keep in mind the transferability of their skills to nontraditional settings.

Since OTs carry an eclectic background of skills, I realized that we should utilize all of them if we can, even if it means working in a nontraditional setting. There is no reason for us as OTs to limit where and how we work when we have such a wide range of skills.

One thing that could not be anticipated was the interviewee's reaction to the idea of occupational therapy in his or her setting. Luckily, the overall reaction to all of the students was positive. The warm reception fueled the enthusiasm to move out into the community as an employment possibility.

. . . the key informant was very eager to learn the information I had to share about OT. He was open and enthusiastic to my idea which only fueled my own enthusiasm.

The students were in situations that demanded they articulate OT services within the particular setting. The definition of OT had to be tailored to the setting and clientele, and translated into the discipline of the key informant. The student had to have a clear idea of their own skills prior to the interview. Information about the agency was investigated beforehand and the instructor was available to coach the student to visualize how OT would fit into the new environment.

This strengthened our creativity and resourcefulness skills and allowed us to get out into the community. Most importantly, I truly had to understand what OT is to effectively complete this assignment (for better or worse) and to understand what OT has to offer the world.

Transition

A third theme that emerged was one of *transition* as students synthesized their learning into a job of their own creation. The words "refreshing," "celebration," and "exciting" were incorporated into the student responses, indicating it was a positive experience for them to culminate two intensive years of study.

> It is refreshing to wrap up our OT curriculum with a fresh and creative outlook on emerging markets for OT.

> I think we are all very excited to enter this career after discovering so many new exciting areas of OT to explore.

> This project is a celebration of what OT can do and in an unstable job market this project provides hope for the future of occupational therapy.

Students were enthusiastic in their responses to fellow presenters. As a summarizing event, it brought closure to the course on an optimistic note.

> It is excellent practice to face some real OT issues. OTs are having to look into emerging markets to assure the future of OT.

> It was a good way to bring all of our coursework together.

> It tied everything we learned together and forced me to reflect on the curriculum and what I have learned the past two years.

EVALUATING PRESENTATIONS

Objective 3, articulating OT services, was measured by rating how well students could articulate the role of OT in their presentations in class, the paired-student response, and by gauging the agency response to each student as subjectively reported by the student interviewers. Out of 23 settings, two students felt that the key informant was reluctant to consider OT as a viable service option. Of the two, one setting's concern was drawing the income necessary to support an OT practitioner due to the fee-for-service arrangement. Only one student was not graciously accommodated at the first attempt to set up an interview and, upon a second attempt, set up a successful interview with another agency staff member. One site offered the student a position upon graduation, and three sites invited the student to return and seek a position in the agency.

The instructor of the course rated the student presentations as very good to excellent. All the students demonstrated exceptional ability in articulating the role of the OT in the new environment. A few of the presentations had weaker areas in program description and/or client assessment of need.

FOCUS GROUP

The focus group, a standard part of all course evaluations, was conducted with 22 students present to gain a sense of how the assignment could be improved for subsequent student groups. The students were asked to respond to open-ended questions about the texts, course content, and assignments. The consensus was the assignment was effective in meeting the objectives of the course. There were some suggestions for improvement:

- The paper was time consuming at the end of the semester and redundant with preparation for the presentation. The written portion that the students felt was important to retain was the job description. The other pieces of the written report seemed to repeat skills already evaluated through other coursework such as the agency needs assessment and program description.
- Require that the students use a multimedia projector in their presentations. The students who used a power point program reported that it was a good experience and that the presentation motivated them to develop the skill. The students who used other presentation methods reported they would have liked to learn the computer skill.
- Some of the students would have liked more time for the presentation. Although the information was covered adequately in a 15-minute presentation, a couple of students who chose more complex sites would have appreciated more time.

DISCUSSION

With the expanded definition of OT service, the debate surfaced regarding the extent to which the scope of OT practice could or should extend before it is no longer occupational therapy. Some students recognized the uncertainty brought on by more fluid definitions and felt the profession would be creating turf wars if it extended the domain of practice too far. Redefining occupation to well populations in the form of lifestyle redesign and stress management programs presented challenges in creating the job descriptions. The question consistently was posed concerning the uniqueness of OT or the "edge" OT brings beyond the other professions who serve in a parallel capacity. The students began to ask: what is the "activity" intervention and where are the skill sources for that position? Questions regarding licensure and domain of practice were discussed. The dialogue throughout the process seemed to generate thoughtful questions even when answers were not readily available. Discussing the uncertainty in the students' future job searches appeared to diminish anxieties when paired with the experience of going into the field and doing a hands-on, real-world probe of the possibilities.

Two portions of the assignment seem to enhance the learning experience in ways that former assignments did not achieve. The first was the initial step. It was student-centered learning with the starting point being the unique skills and talents of the individual learner. It is difficult to tailor learning in a professional program where, often, the content drives the process. Oftentimes, the students' unique interests cannot be served within the criteria established for grading individual assignments. The motivational factor seemed to be elevated for all students as they were given permission to express their individuality through their work. The real test results of the assignment will be to survey the students after graduation to see if they pursued work in the area of their choice or even the site they investigated for the project.

The other enhancement was the real-world application. With former assignments, students struggled with uncertainty in creating hypothetical clinics or conceptualized programs void of first-hand experience. Because they had "been there," student presentations had a dimension of confidence extending from a security in their own knowledge base that was not observed other years. They were able to field questions during the presentation with an added maturity, drawing from actual experience.

There are limitations to the management project. It is an investment of time, both on the part of the instructor and the student. In creating learning experiences, the highest payoff is desired for the time and energy invested. Not all curricula can support the magnitude of such a project within the existing curricular format nor have the options of diverse community agencies that are present in larger metropolitan areas.

The management project may not serve the students in the future due to changing markets and reimbursement systems. There are certain elements that will serve the learning process but other portions may find their own obsolescence. The learning experiences are designed to meet the needs of the present students, but may be challenged to change as the needs change for future cohorts. The objectives—to see the future job as a good fit with their skills and interests, to build confidence in translating academic learning to real-world practice, and to articulate the services of the profession—are independent of time, but the experiences are in real-world time. Continued evaluation of curricular projects is an ongoing need in a professional program that strives to serve its students with innovation.

REFERENCES

American Occupational Therapy Association (1996). *Managed care: An occupational therapy sourcebook.* Bethesda, MD: AOTA, Inc.

American Occupational Therapy Association (1996). *The occupational therapy manager.* Bethesda, MD: AOTA, Inc.

American Occupational Therapy Association (1999). *Occupational therapy services for children and youth under the individuals with disabilities education act (IDEA), 2nd edition.* Bethesda, MD: AOTA, Inc.

Boyd, S. D. (1995). Practicing short leaps: Unleashing your creativity in managing people and resources. Minnesota Association of Homes for the Aging conference presentation. Feb. 9, 1995.

Christiansen, C. H. (1975). Attitudes of graduates. *American Journal of Occupational Therapy, 29(6),* 355.

Foto, M. (1998). The health care revolution: A catalyst for professional evolution. *American Journal of Occupational Therapy, 52(4),* 247.

Jacobs, K. (2000). Under renovation: Incorporating change. *American Journal of Occupational Therapy, 54(5),* 457.

Loukas, K. M. (2000). Emerging models of innovative community-based occupational practice. *OT Practice, 5(14),* 9.

Miles, M. B. (1997). *Qualitative Data Analysis.* London: Sage Publications, Inc.

Steib, P. (1999). Survey: Most practitioners holding their own. *OT Week, March 11, 1999.*

The Partnering Model:
Occupational Therapy Assistant
and Occupational Therapy Students
Working Together

Carol R. Scheerer, EdD, OTR/L

SUMMARY. Establishing a partnering relationship between the occupational therapy assistant (OTA) and the occupational therapist (OT) is imperative in order to create an optimal working environment and deliver effective client care. A developmental model that provides students with opportunities to practice such a relationship has been used by an OTA and OT program in southwestern Ohio. This developmental Partnering Model gives students an opportunity to interact, work as teams, and collaborate during their educational experience. Each aspect of the model provides students with experiential learning opportunities. Educators will serve their OTA and OT students well in providing opportunities for them to develop and practice the skills they will need to create an optimal working environment and deliver effective client care as occupational therapy practitioners. *[Article copies available for a fee from The Haworth Document Delivery Service: 1-800-HAWORTH. E-mail address: <getinfo@haworthpressinc.com> Website: <http://www.HaworthPress.com> © 2001 by The Haworth Press, Inc. All rights reserved.]*

Carol R. Scheerer, Assistant Professor, is affiliated with Xavier University, Department of Occupational Therapy, 3800 Victory Parkway, Cincinnati, OH 45207-7341 (E-mail: scheerer@xu.edu).

[Haworth co-indexing entry note]: "The Partnering Model: Occupational Therapy Assistant and Occupational Therapy Students Working Together." Scheerer, Carol R. Co-published simultaneously in *Occupational Therapy in Health Care* (The Haworth Press, Inc.) Vol. 15, No. 1/2, 2001, pp. 193-208; and: *Education for Occupational Therapy in Health Care: Strategies for the New Millennium* (eds: Patricia Crist, and Marjorie Scaffa) The Haworth Press, Inc., 2001, pp. 193-208. Single or multiple copies of this article are available for a fee from The Haworth Document Delivery Service [1-800-HAWORTH, 9:00 a.m. - 5:00 p.m. (EST). E-mail address: getinfo@haworthpressinc.com].

KEYWORDS. Education, occupational therapy practitioners, collaboration

INTRODUCTION AND PURPOSE

Occupational therapists are trained to work as members of a team. Ironically, at times, they have difficulty working effectively with the team member with whom they are most closely aligned, the occupational therapy assistant. It is believed that the combined skills of the practitioners are greater than the sum of their separate skills (COTA and OTR Education Unit Task Force, 1997; Glantz & Richman, 1997; Holmes & Black, 1995), yet the required supervision of the occupational therapy assistant (OTA) by the occupational therapist (OT) can present a challenge. There has been evidence of role confusion between the two with neither practitioner completely understanding the responsibilities of the other (Coleman & Riley, 1997; Egan, 1992). Additional strain has occurred because the OT has not always been adequately trained in supervision. At times, the relationship between the two has been guarded (Egan, 1992). Traditionally, the OTA and OT have been trained at two-year and four-year programs, respectively, with the OT education recently upgraded to entry-level masters preparation. This broadening of the educational differences certainly has the potential to increase the confusion. As a means of preventing such an occurrence, the OTA and OT must develop a better understanding of their roles. Educators carry the responsibility of preparing practitioners for their future career roles. As the level of preparedness between the practitioners widens, this is an opportune time for educators to focus on promoting cooperation and partnering between the OTA and OT.

The purpose of this article is to share with the reader a Partnering Model used in two educational settings to facilitate the OTA/OT relationship. It is anticipated that the sharing of experienced educational activities and techniques used in this model may serve as a springboard for other educational programs across the country. Implementing educationally sound experiential activities that meet students' needs will enhance student learning and the ability to develop effective partnering skills.

REVIEW OF THE LITERATURE

Effectively working together as OTA and OT partners is not a skill that should be left to chance. This skill needs to be developed (AOTA, 2000b) and cultivated. As Kielhofner (1997) suggests, when a behavior becomes a habit it can then be used routinely and automatically. Partnering between the OT/OTA team needs to become a habit so that future practitioners can use it as part of their daily occupation. To develop this partnering habit, practice in doing so needs to be embedded in the educational curriculum of future occupational therapy practitioners.

The principles in the OT Code of Ethics (2000) (AOTA, 2000a) address an occupational therapy practitioner's supervision responsibilities as do state licensure laws and regulations. The *Standards for an Accredited Educational Program for the Occupational Therapy Assistant* (ACOTE of the AOTA, 1999b) mandate articulation of the importance of the professional relationship. The *Standards for an Accredited Educational Program for the Occupational Therapist* (ACOTE of the AOTA, 1999a) emphasize the development of OT skills in supervision and collaboration. These standards direct the curriculum content for OTA and OT educational programs. A curriculum can be considered a means of "aiding and abetting a learner" (Bruner, 1996, p. 116) and is a work in progress directing the behavior of future OT practitioners. "The curriculum creates the future" (Yerxa, 1998, p. 366). Placing the development of partnering skills in the curriculum will better prepare practitioners for their future career roles.

Much has been written about the needed cooperation and partnership between the OTA/OT team. Understanding each other's role in the partnership and on the interdisciplinary team is critical (Black, 1996; Egan, 1992; Sands, 1998). Mutual respect and trust are often considered the cornerstones of the relationship (AOTA, 2000b; Black, 1996; Campbell, 1998; Sands, 1998). Ongoing communication is a key (Black, 1996; Egan, 1992; Herzberg, 1994). Teamwork is important (Herzberg, 1994) and supervisory skills for the OT are critical (Lawrence, 1993; Hawkins, 1991) with both practitioners taking responsibility and benefiting from the supervisory process (Campbell, 1998). Black (1996) advocates for a strong OTA/OT relationship. She draws from Covey (1991), who suggests that in a strong team, when the goals are the same, the differences in roles are used as strengths. As the needed attributes of the partnership are put into play, the clients with whom the OTA and OT provide services benefit by receiving efficient, effective, and cost-effective care (Glanz & Richman, 1997). A strong relationship between the two professionals increases the potential for job satisfaction and decreases the incidence of job burnout (Glantz & Richman, 1997). Furthermore, as the OTA role expands (Cottrell, 2000), the field of occupational therapy benefits as development of the strengths of both practitioners contributes to growth of the profession.

Specific examples of cooperation and partnering have been reported in the literature. OTA/OT collaborative educational initiatives have been used in academia (Coleman & Riley, 1997; COTA and OTR Education Unit Task Force,

1997; Holmes & Black, 1995), in fieldwork settings (Higgins, 1998), and in practice settings (DiMatties, 1995; Glantz & Richman, 1997). The COTA and OTR Educational Unit Task Force (1997) recommends that OTA and OT students meet face-to-face to interact, communicate, and collaborate in preparation for their career roles. Holmes and Black (1995) recommend that to lay the foundation for respectful partnerships, OTA and OT students have direct contact with each other, collaboratively learn content, and incorporate supervision theory in their curriculum. Clearly, OTA/OT partnering initiatives are needed to prepare students for their future career as occupational therapy practitioners.

METHODS AND RESULTS

Faculty from an OTA and an OT program located at separate facilities in the same large, urban metropolitan area of a Midwestern city have worked together to create initiatives that promote partnering between their students. The initiatives followed an "OTA/OT Partnering Model," a curricular developmental hierarchy developed by the two schools. Students were initially brought together to interact, they then functioned together as a team, and finally they worked together in a collaborative manner. The details of this OTA/OT Partnering Model used during the school year 1999-2000 will be further described.

Interaction Level: Session One

At the Interaction level (see Figure 1), two, two-hour joint sessions were held in the fall semester between the first-year students in both programs. The topic of these sessions was role delineation. To become familiar with the content, students were given study questions taken from Kief and Scheerer (2001) (in press at the time) to complete prior to the session. Neistadt and Crepeau (1998), Ryan (1995) and the Official Documents of AOTA (AOTA, 1998a) were used as texts from which the students could find answers to these study questions. The OTA program hosted the first two-hour session with breakfast provided by the students. Name tags were donned and faculty members introduced. Students were divided into small groups of approximately two occupational therapy assistant students (OTAS) and two occupational therapy students (OTS).

The groups were given a copy of each school's curriculum and asked to review content identifying similarities and differences. A study sheet guided the students to ask each other additional personal-related information so they would have a chance to get to know each other. The class reconvened for large

FIGURE 1. Developmental Hierarchy of the OTA/OT Partnering Model

Level III: Collaboration **(Collaborative research groups)** ↑ ↑ **Level II: Teamwork** **(Joint assignments/projects)** ↑ ↑ **Level I: Interaction** **(Joint sessions/activities)**
OTA/OT PARTNERING MODEL

group discussion, and the instructors recorded on the chalkboard the most notable similarities and differences between the two programs. Students could see the overlapping areas of normal development, occupation and occupational analysis, disabling conditions, and intervention techniques, as well as anatomy and physiology. The notable differences included the theory-based information, the in-depth look at frames of reference used to guide practice, as well as the emphasis on the evaluation process and research in the OT program.

For the second activity of the first session, students were again divided into OTA/OT groups of four or five, with each group assigned a section of the *Standards of Practice for Occupational Therapy (Standards)* (AOTA, 1998b). Each group was assigned a section of the *Standards* and illustrated on chart paper a visual representation or mind map of that section. Role delineations of each section were emphasized. After completion of the drawing, each group shared with the entire group the interpretation of their drawing as they helped their peers visually see each step of the OT process as well as understand the definitions and roles contained therein.

For the final activity of the first session, students remained in their previously formed groups. The instructors read a short description of a client or occurrence related to the different *Standards* (AOTA, 1998b). The groups then identified which standard addressed the contrived scenario. Points were awarded for the teams as students identified the linkage between the scenario and the specific standard. The team with the greatest number of points was awarded a prize token (tablet of paper for each person). To close the session, a tour of the facility was conducted. The OT students familiarized themselves with the OTA students' educational environment as they walked through the classroom and lab areas used by the OTA students.

Interaction Level: Session Two

The second session was held several weeks later and began in a similar fashion to the first. Students were given additional role delineation study questions (Kief & Scheerer, 2001), using the previously named texts, and asked to complete them prior to the session. The OT institution hosted this session, with breakfast again being provided by the students. As before, name tags were distributed and the faculty members introduced. The entire group was then divided into smaller groups of two to three OTA and OT students. Each group was given one of four case studies taken from Kief and Scheerer (2001). Using an outline of the *Standards* (AOTA, 1998b), each group determined which aspects of the OT process could be completed by the OTA and the OT for the client in their particular case study. Students then used the chart that delineates the roles of the OTA and OT in *The Guide to Occupational Therapy Practice* (Moyers, 1999) to check the accuracy of their work. All students reconvened for a discussion, with small groups articulating their role delineation rationale to the rest of the class.

The second activity for the session consisted of a Scattergories™-type game (Kief & Scheerer, 2001). Students were divided into ten teams. Each team had two minutes to generate a list of one-word descriptors of an "ideal" OTA/OT relationship. Each group then shared their descriptors with the class in a round-robin fashion. Points were awarded each time a team contributed a new descriptor to the list. The final list consisted of 100 descriptor words, including respect, friendship, support, consideration, interdependent, productive, and encouraging. Again, a token prize was awarded to the winning team (pens from the host institution). At the end of the session, the students toured the OT classroom and lab facilities. In a reciprocal manner, the OTA students could see where the OT students spent their educational time during the day.

At a later date, faculty of the respective institutions had their classes divide into small groups to generate a list of ongoing methods and/or activities that would assist in developing and enhancing relationships between the students of the two programs. Students were asked to list goals for the activities as well (Kief & Scheerer, 2001). Examples of goals generated were those of working together as an OTA/OT team; establishing a comfortable, friendly, respectful, and helpful relationship between students; and developing networking skills. To meet those goals, among the ideas given were having social times outside of class, exchanging guest speakers, joining the student clubs for functions, and having students work together on joint projects or research. The faculty members of the institutions shared these ideas for consideration.

During these separate class sessions, informal evaluative feedback was also solicited from the OTA students and OT students. Students commented that the sessions were helpful in establishing the OTA/OT relationship. They felt it was a good idea to get the two groups of students together, and the word game was especially appreciated, as it served as a tension reducer. Students also had several suggestions to enhance future learning activities. For example, they suggested re-ordering the activities presented so that emphasis would first be placed on the type of ideal relationship and that strengths and similarities would be the initial foci. This could then serve as a foundation for future activities and emphasize the importance of relationships as a foundation for partnering.

Teamwork Level

The second step in the developmental model is that of Teamwork (see Figure 1). To promote teamwork, a joint assignment was given to the classes at the two schools. Second-semester, first-year OT students were paired with second-year OTA students to complete this joint assignment that was part of a group process course for the OT students and part of a therapeutic media course for the OTA students. Students were assigned partners by the instructors and worked in small groups of two to three OTA and OT students. For the joint assignment, students were required to observe a local support group of their choice. After observing the support group, students were required to write a paper identifying group norms, member roles, and observations related to group process and content. The students were also required to describe how such a support group might relate to their future role as an OT practitioner. Students wrote the paper as a team effort. The final aspect of the assignment required each individual to add a separate paragraph reflecting on the teamwork and collaborative experience. This provided an opportunity for both parties to give feedback to the other team member(s). Following the writing of the paper, students gave a class presentation to their peers at their respective schools to explain and describe their experiences. Consequently, all students benefited from hearing about the types of support groups to which they may refer their future clients. The respective institution's faculty graded the papers and presentations.

Simultaneously, another teamwork project (Kief & Scheerer, 2001) was in process that involved the first-year OT students and the second-year OTA students. Students from both institutions opted to complete this project as a course elective. They were given a scenario that included the particulars of a case-study client. For this case study, the OTs selected the assessments to be completed, while goal writing, intervention planning, and implementation were completed, jointly by the OTAs and OTs. Notes on the simulated tasks and activities of the OT process were sent between the two parties via postal mail, e-mail, and fax, with the OTs co-signing the OTA's notes. Three groups of students completed this one-semester project.

Collaboration Level

The final tier of the OTA/OT Partnering Model (see Figure 1) provided students an opportunity to develop the skill of Collaboration. OTA students served as "research assistants" to senior OT students who were required to complete a research project in conjunction with a faculty tutor and/or a clinical tutor. Groups of OT students determined whether they needed a research assistant and then posted, via an Internet online message system, the nature of their project and the anticipated duties of the assistant. The second-year OTA students reviewed their options and signed up for a one-hour elective course selecting the research project that aligned with their interest. Initially, out of the fourteen OT research groups, six of them requested and were assigned a research assistant. As time went on and busy schedules factored in, four of the OTA students dropped the course. The remaining two teams carried out their research projects. For these two projects, the OT students supervised the OTA students who assisted with data collection and/or entering data in the computer for analysis. One group used the collaborative relationship productively and successfully and included the OTA student in their presentation at the Spring Research Symposium (a formal presentation to faculty, students, and clinicians in the area). This research team reported that all went well and that the research assistant was very helpful to the overall research process. They further stated it was worth the time and energy needed to make the collaborative process work as they got to know the OTA better as a person, as well as her capabilities and program.

DISCUSSION

This Partnering Model is based on hierarchical joint teaching-learning experiences. Combined sessions were designed to promote better understanding and appreciation of each other's roles between OTA and OT students. The sessions and activities progressed from interactive to teamwork to collaboration. The educational effectiveness of a variety of methods used in these sessions is substantiated in the professional literature.

Research denotes that occupational therapy students want hands-on and active learning (Fisher, 1999). Borich (1996) identifies student engagement in the learning process as a key teaching technique. Good and Brophy (1997) have found students prefer "active" or "doing" assignments which contribute to students' intrinsic motivation. Such engagement was used during all phases of the Partnering Model. At the Interaction level, active learning was evident as students completed drawings together and participated in the educational games. At the Teamwork level, active learning occurred in the writing of the joint paper and in completing the joint support group assignment. At the Collaboration level, it occurred as research roles were first negotiated and then implemented for the final project. The hands-on experience, joint problem solving, and social interaction that occurred with these activities are all documented characteristics of constructivist teaching and learning (Borich, 1996).

Constructivist theory (Steffe & Gale, 1995) suggests that ongoing knowledge is gained by pairing it with previous knowledge learned. Building on a student's previous knowledge, a type of scaffolding or building layer upon layer of knowledge, is seen as an effective teaching technique facilitating student learning (Good & Brophy, 1997). The pre-session study questions provided a foundation for the progression of learning during the joint sessions. Furthermore, "questioning" is one academic tool that supports student learning, and providing questions to the students in advance gave them time to formulate thoughtful answers, a technique tied to effective teaching (Borich, 1996). In this way the questions might be considered a type of "advance organizer" (Good & Brophy, 1997, p. 240), preparing students to know what is expected of them.

In addition to the hands-on activities and study questions, a variety of instructional methods and teaching styles were used, including small group learning, written assignments, and oral presentations. Varying the type of teaching style used meets the needs of more students, as students have a variety of preferred ways of learning. Kolb (1984) identifies four types of learning styles: accommodator, diverger, converger, assimilator. OT students, in particular, are thought to be accommodator learners, as they tend to have a preference to be "concrete" and "experiential" (Katz & Heimann, 1991), showing a preference for hands-on lab practice (Graham & Babola, 1998). Expanding beyond a lecture presentation to a hands-on mode helps students learn by tapping into more than one type of intelligence. Gardner (1983) presents the concept of multiple intelligences, and hands-on activities are aligned with his identified body kinesthetic type of intelligence.

OT students have reported that expressing their own interests and personalities in their work is a beneficial educational strategy (Fisher, 1999). Knowles (1989) suggests that when adult learners are part of the instructional planning, their motivation to learn increases. Good and Brophy (1997) suggest students will value what they are doing when they are given autonomy in educational decisions. Autonomy was given when students selected the support groups they wanted to observe for the joint project assignment. Incorporating the goals and ideas generated by the students after the two joint sessions was a way of using student ideas and contributions. Additionally, self-directed learning facilitates the development of higher-order thinking skills (Borich, 1996).

Occupational therapy students also appreciate the use of visual aids (Fisher, 1999). Perception and retention of material is often improved when visuals are added to text (Bruning, Schraw, & Ronning, 1999). Visuals can also help clarify abstract concepts (Rakes, 1996). Drawing a mind map and explaining the drawing to classmates provided a pictorial way of helping students remember the different aspects of the *Standards*.

Small group work is another effective teaching tool used in this Partnering Model process. It can affect student learning by promoting engagement in the learning process (Borich, 1996). Working together in groups or communities can be energizing (Gabelnick, MacGregor, Matthews, & Smith, 1990) and can actively engage students as well as increase their motivation and learning (Good & Brophy, 1997). Small group work was employed as a teaching tool in all phases of this Partnering Model in joint sessions/activities, in joint assignments/projects, and in collaborative research groups. Similarly, small group games are a way to make small group work more enjoyable. Instructional games have also been suggested as an effective teaching technique (Roberts, 1993). The Scattergories™-type game and *Standards* (AOTA, 1998b) activity are examples of using educational games as part of the learning process.

Occupational therapy students have identified the use of case studies as a helpful teaching tool (Fisher, 1999). Students compared their case study answers regarding role delineation within the OT process to Moyers' (1999) chart delineating the practitioner roles. This exemplifies the technique called "checking for understanding" (Rosenshine & Stevens, 1986, p. 379). This technique is an important part of guided practice, a systematic teacher-directed instructional format that is considered an effective instructional technique.

Occupational therapy students have also identified student presentations as an effective teaching tool (Fisher, 1999). As one student stated, "Students teaching each other–the ultimate test of knowledge" (Graham & Babola, 1998, p. 200). This Partnering Model provided students multiple opportunities to give presentations, such as when students presented their "mind map," when they explained the rationale for use of their case study, when they presented their support group project to their peers, and when the OTA/OT group presented at the research symposium.

"Reflection" has been shown to be a valuable tool for both clinicians and students. Schon (1987) talks of the reflective practitioner and the importance of reflection in the learning process. Similarly, Mattingly and Fleming (1994) see reflection as an important part of the clinical reasoning skills needed by occupational therapists. Reflection was incorporated when requiring a reflective part of the assignment for the support group project. Bruning, Schraw, and

Ronning (1999) suggest that students' reflection upon their own learning nurtures cognitive growth. Woods (1994) sees self-assessment as an important component of a student's ability to improve interpersonal skills. Interpersonal skill reflection was part of the OTA/OT joint assignment.

Strong interpersonal skills were needed at all levels of the Partnering Model. An interpersonal skill, that of being able to get along with others, has been shown to be important in the workplace (Elder & Nick, 1997) and in fieldwork experiences (Tickle-Degnen, 1998). Students had an opportunity to socialize during the refreshment phases and further developed this skill when completing support group projects as well as the research project. Pre-assignment of partners by faculty for the support group assignment simulated a real-life scenario where a person does not necessarily get to select his/her co-workers but rather needs to learn to get along with whomever is on the team (Collier & O'Conner, 1998). Flexibility and adaptability, desired clinical characteristics (Herzberg, 1994), and aspects of professional behavior (Bossers, Kernaghan, Hodgins, Merla, O'Conner, & Van Kessel, 1999) were crucial aspects involved with negotiating meeting and writing times for the support group assignment. These professional behaviors were also used during data collection, analysis, and presentation practice for the collaborative research teams. An optimal working environment can better be realized when the interpersonal skills of team members are strong.

Interpersonal skills are further strengthened by developing effective communication skills. Opportunities to develop communication skills were provided throughout the assignments. Communication has been identified as a skill needed to participate as an effective interdisciplinary team member (Foto, 1997), a means of facilitating effective supervision (Sands, 1998), and a needed skill in the clinic (Collier & O'Conner, 1998). Effective communication was required in the Interaction phase in order for the paired groups to work together. The competition of the games facilitated communication among members as they determined the aspect of the *Standards* (AOTA, 1998b) represented by the scenario as well as the characteristics that described the OTA/OT relationship. Effective communication was vital in coordinating the schedules for selecting and attending the support groups, in completing the teamwork project, in writing the paper for the joint assignment as well as in completing the research process.

A critical component of communication skills is the ability to effectively give and receive feedback. This ability has been identified as an important skill in the OTA/OT partnership (Black, 1996). Feedback can be used to promote continuing competence in practitioners (Youngstrom, 1998). The ability to give and receive feedback was practiced when students reflected upon the interpersonal skills used during completion of the support group assignment.

Finally, using activities designed around the Partnering Model levels of Interaction, Teamwork, and Collaboration throughout the curriculum helped provide students with real-world tasks. Borich (1996) defines real-world tasks as authentic tasks. Authentic educational activities contribute to a student's motivation (Good & Brophy, 1997). The real world requires the OTA and OT to interact, work as teams, and collaborate. Additionally, the real world requires some level of OTA supervision by the OT. Practice in supervision was seen when the collaborative research group negotiated roles and worked as partners. The OTAs served as a research assistant to the OTs who served as a beginning research investigator allowing both of them to assume the roles and functions outlined as entry-level research competencies (Academic Development Committee, Research Advisory Council, American Occupational Therapy Foundation, 2000). Practicing supervision prepares students for real-life partnerships. Practicing the Interaction, Teamwork, and Collaboration used in the Partnering Model gave students an opportunity to sample the experiences they will encounter as future practitioners.

CONCLUSION

The developmental hierarchy of the OTA/OT Partnering Model represents a constructivist approach to learning and was designed to meet the varied learning styles of students. Each layer built on the students' prior knowledge and experiences. It is anticipated OTA and OT students will be able to work more effectively as team members since they previously interacted with each other; they will be able to work collaboratively because they have learned the delineations of their roles, the type of relationship needed, and have experienced working in teams; they will be able to form partnerships because they have engaged in supervisory and collaborative experiences. The educational activities presented facilitated effective construction of knowledge not only through "hands-on" learning but what Danielson (1996) refers to as "minds-on" learning. Minds were engaged while practicing partnering, an authentic and real-life task.

Practicing interaction, teamwork, and collaboration as students should promote a lifetime habit of partnering as practitioners. Yerxa, Clark, Frank, Jackson, Parham, Pierce, Stein, and Zemke (1989) suggest occupation enables people to contribute to society. Similarly, the occupation of partnering will allow OTA/OT students to contribute not only to society but also to the health and well-being of their clients and profession. Educators can serve their students well to use and build upon the OTA/OT Partnering Model as they design instruction to give future occupational therapy practitioners an opportunity to develop and practice the skills they will need to create an optimal working environment ultimately delivering more effective client care.

Further development of instructional methods expanding on this developmental hierarchy model is warranted. Effective teaching can be realized by including experiential learning activities at each level of the Partnering Model. Looking more specifically at the outcomes of each level of this model, for example, looking at the multiple benefits of engaging in a collaborative research process, will garner support beyond the current literature-based evidence provided.

AUTHOR NOTE

The author would like to acknowledge Cindy Kief, Coordinator/Instructor, Cincinnati State Technical and Community College, and Claudia Miller, Program Chairperson, Cincinnati State Technical and Community College, for their continuous collaboration and teamwork in developing this partnering model. Further acknowledgment goes to Joanne Phillips Estes, Department Chairperson and Assistant Professor, Xavier University, and Georganna Miller, Academic Fieldwork Coordinator and Faculty, Xavier University, for their support and assistance in reviewing this manuscript.

This manuscript was completed in partial fulfillment of a doctorate degree in education from the University of Cincinnati. The contents of this manuscript were presented at the Ohio Occupational Therapy Association Conference held in Toledo, October, 2000 (co-presenters were Claudia Miller, MHS, OTR/L, and Cindy Kief, COTA/L, AP). Additionally, an abstract of the contents of this manuscript has been accepted for a short course presentation at the American Occupational Therapy Association Conference, 2001, in Philadelphia.

REFERENCES

Academic Development Committee, Research Advisory Council, American Occupational Therapy Foundation. (2000). Levels of research competence across the profession of occupational therapy. *American Journal of Occupational Therapy, 54* (3), 344-346.

Accreditation Council for Occupational Therapy Education of the American Occupational Therapy Association. (1999a). Standards for an accredited educational program for the occupational therapist. *American Journal of Occupational Therapy, 53* (6), 575-582.

Accreditation Council for Occupational Therapy Education of the American Occupational Therapy Association. (1999b). Standards for an accredited educational program for the occupational therapy assistant. *American Occupational Therapy, 53* (6), 583-589.

American Occupational Therapy Association. (1998a). *Reference manual of the official documents of the American Occupational Therapy Association*. Bethesda, MD: Author.

American Occupational Therapy Association. (1998b). Standards of practice for occupational therapy. *American Journal of Occupational Therapy, 52* (10), 866-869.

American Occupational Therapy Association. (2000a). Occupational therapy code of ethics (2000). *American Journal of Occupational Therapy, 54* (6), 614-616.

American Occupational Therapy Association. (2000b). *OTA information packet.* Bethesda, MD: Author.

Black, T. (1996). COTAs and OTRs as partners and teams. *OT Practice, 1* (3), 42-47.

Borich, G. D. (1996). *Effective teaching methods* (3rd ed.). Englewood Cliffs, NJ: Prentice Hall.

Bossers, A., Kernaghan, J., Hodgins, L., Merla, L., O'Conner, C., & Kessel, M. V. (1999). Defining and developing professionalism. *Canadian Journal of Occupational Therapy, 66* (3), 116-121.

Bruner, J. (1996). *The culture of education.* Cambridge, MA: Harvard University Press.

Bruning, R. H., Schraw, G. J., & Ronning, R. R. (1999). *Cognitive psychology and instruction* (3rd ed.). Upper Saddle River, NJ: Prentice Hall.

Campbell, K. J. (1998). OTA focus: Forging OTA-OT partnerships that work. *OT Week, 12* (21), 10.

Coleman, S., & Riley, M. (1997). OT/OTA education–Beginning the collaborative relationship. *OT Practice, 2* (4), 55-57.

Collier, G. F., & O'Conner, L. (1998). Increasing efficiency and effectiveness in Level II Fieldwork–Collaborative supervision, real-life skills. *OT Practice, 3* (4), 46-48.

COTA and OTR Education Unit Task Force. (1997). *COTA and OTR education unit.* Bethesda, MD: American Occupational Therapy Association.

Cottrell, R. P. F. (2000). COTA education and professional development: A historical review. *American Journal of Occupational Therapy, 54* (4), 407-412.

Covey, S. R. (1991). *Principle-centered leadership.* New York: Simon and Schuster.

Danielson, C. (1996). *Enhancing professional practice: A framework for teaching.* Alexandria, VA: Association for Supervision and Curriculum Development.

DiMatties, M. E. (1995). The occupational therapist-certified occupational therapy assistant partnership in a public school. *School System Special Interest Section Newsletter, 2* (3), 1-2.

Egan, M. (1992). Focus COTAs–COTAs and OTRs in conversation: Respecting the relationship. *OT Week, 6,* 14-15.

Elder, Jr., O. C., & Nick, T. G. (1997). Moving toward a core curriculum in schools of the allied health professions: Knowledge and skills considered important by department chairs in four disciplines. *Journal of Allied Health, 26* (2), 51-56.

Fisher, G. S. (1999). A study of successful educational strategies in three entry-level graduate programs. *Occupational Therapy in Health Care, 12* (1), 17-31.

Foto, M. (1997). Nationally speaking–Preparing occupational therapists for the year 2000: The impact of managed care on education and training. *American Journal of Occupational Therapy, 51* (2), 88-90.

Gabelnick, F., MacGregor, J., Matthews, R. S., & Smith, B. L. (1990). Teaching in learning communities. *New Directions for Teaching and Learning, 41,* 53-60.

Gardner, H. (1983). *Frames of mind: The theory of multiple intelligences.* New York: Basic Books.

Glantz, C. H., & Richman, N. (1997). OTR-COTA collaboration in home health: Roles and supervisory issues. *American Journal of Occupational Therapy, 51* (6), 446-452.

Good, T. L., & Brophy, J. E. (1997). *Looking in classrooms* (7th ed.). New York: Longman.

Graham, C., & Babola, K. (1998). Needs assessment of non-traditional students in physical and occupational therapy programs. *Journal of Allied Health, 27* (4), 196-201.

Hawkins, T. R. (1991). Supervising the occupational therapy assistant student. *Administration and Management Special Interest Section Newsletter, 7* (1), 1-2.

Herzberg, G. L. (1994). The successful fieldwork student: Supervisor perceptions. *American Journal of Occupational Therapy, 48* (9), 817-823.

Higgins, S. M. (1998). The OT/OTA collaborative model of fieldwork education. *OT Practice, 3* (10), 41-44.

Holmes, C., & Black, T. (1995). Modifying the occupational therapy managerial structure to improve the role of the certified occupational therapy assistant. *Education Special Interest Section Newsletter, 5* (3), 1-3.

Katz, N., & Heimann, N. (1991). Learning style of students and practitioners in five health professions. *Occupational Therapy Journal of Research, 11* (4), 238-244.

Kief, C., & Scheerer, C. (2001). *Clinical competencies in occupational therapy.* Upper Saddle River, NJ: Prentice Hall.

Kielhofner, G. (1997). *Conceptual foundations of occupational therapy* (2nd ed.). Philadelphia: F. A. Davis.

Knowles, M. S. (1989). *The making of an adult educator: An autobiographical journey.* San Francisco: Jossey-Bass.

Kolb, D. A. (1984). *Experiential learning: Experience as the source of learning and development.* Englewood Cliffs, NJ: Prentice-Hall.

Lawrence, L. J. (1993). A practical application of role delineation for the certified occupational therapy assistant. *Physical Disabilities Special Interest Section Newsletter, 16* (4), 2-4.

Mattingly, C., & Fleming, M. H. (1994). *Clinical reasoning: Forms of inquiry in a therapeutic practice.* Philadelphia: F. A. Davis.

Moyers, P. A. (1999). The guide to occupational therapy practice. *American Journal of Occupational Therapy, 53* (3), 247-322.

Neistadt, M. E., & Crepeau, E. B. (1998). *Willard and Spackman's occupational therapy* (9th ed.). Philadelphia: Lippincott.

Rakes, G. C. (1996). Visuals in instructional design. *Performance and Instruction, 35* (3), 30-32.

Roberts, A. E. (1993). An evaluation of the effectiveness of educational gaming as a teaching method for therapists. *British Journal of Occupational Therapy, 56* (10), 371-375.

Rosenshine, B., & Stevens, R. (1986). Teaching functions. In M. C. Wittrock (Ed.), *Handbook of research on teaching* (pp. 376-391). Washington DC: American Educational Research Association.

Ryan, S. E. (1995). *Practice issues in occupational therapy: Intraprofessional team building*. Thorofare, NJ: Slack.

Sands, M. (1998). Practitioners' perspectives on the occupational therapist and occupational therapy assistant partnership. In M. E. Neistadt & E. B. Crepeau (Eds.), *Willard and Spackman's occupational therapy* (9th ed., pp. 83-89). Philadelphia: Lippincott.

Schon, D. A. (1987). *Educating the reflective practitioner*. San Francisco: Jossey-Bass.

Steffe, L., & Gale, J. (Eds.). (1995). *Constructivism in education*. Hillsdale, NJ: Erlbaum.

Tickle-Degnen, L. (1998). Working well with others: The prediction of students' clinical performance. *American Journal of Occupational Therapy, 52* (2), 133-142.

Woods, D. R. (1994). Problem solving and interpersonal skills. *Journal of College Science Teaching, 23* (6), 380-381.

Yerxa, E. J. (1998). Occupation: The keystone of a curriculum for a self-defined profession. *American Journal of Occupational Therapy, 52* (5), 365-371.

Yerxa, E. J., Clark, F., Frank, G., Jackson, J., Parham, D., Pierce, D., Stein, C., & Zemke, R. (1989). An introduction to occupational science, a foundation for occupational therapy in the 21st century. *Occupational Therapy in Health Care, 6*, 1-17.

Youngstrom, M. J. (1998). Evolving competence in the practitioner role. *American Journal of Occupational Therapy, 52* (9), 716-720.

Reflections on Education and Learning in Occupational Therapy for the 21st Century

Charlotte Brasic Royeen, PhD, OTR, FAOTA

Because working with clients and their families has an educational component embedded within it, education has always been a focus of occupational therapy. And, just as occupational therapy has changed over the years, so, too, education has changed. The purpose of this essay is to reflect upon what some of these changes in education have been, relate them to occupational therapy education and, based upon this reflection, set priorities needing to be addressed in occupational therapy education for the 21st century. This article reveals many more different issues in education than identified by Grant just 10 years ago (Grant, 1991)!

Charlotte Brasic Royeen is Chairperson, Education Special Interest Section, and recent Chair, Commission on Education, American Occupational Therapy Association. She is also Associate Dean for Research, and Professor in Occupational Therapy, School of Pharmacy and Allied Health Professions, Creighton University, 2500 California Plaza, Omaha, NE 68178 (E-mail: croyeen@creighton.edu).

[Haworth co-indexing entry note]: "Reflections on Education and Learning in Occupational Therapy for the 21st Century." Royeen, Charlotte Brasic. Co-published simultaneously in *Occupational Therapy in Health Care* (The Haworth Press, Inc.) Vol. 15, No. 1/2, 2001, pp. 209-213; and: *Education for Occupational Therapy in Health Care: Strategies for the New Millennium* (eds: Patricia Crist, and Marjorie Scaffa) The Haworth Press, Inc., 2001, pp. 209-213. Single or multiple copies of this article are available for a fee from The Haworth Document Delivery Service [1-800-HAWORTH, 9:00 a.m. - 5:00 p.m. (EST). E-mail address: getinfo@haworthpressinc.com].

CHANGES IN EDUCATION

In the past twenty years, education overall has been revolutionized due to a variety of factors. The most important of these factors are:

• Instructional technology,
• A shift in focus from education to learning, and
• An increased recognition of the need for interdisciplinary collaboration.

Each of these will be discussed in turn.

Instructional Technology. The advent of the Internet, Internet 2, cheaper and more portable computers, and the maturation of Generation X, the first generation to have been raised in a multimedia stream of consciousness, has created a "Brave New World" in education. In spite of whatever attitudes, values, and beliefs any of us hold about technology in education, educational change is here (Baldwin, 1998)! Not only is it here, but also technology in education is forcing a change in the usual and customary ways of operating universities, businesses, and just about every aspect of our lives. Nontraditional education used to mean night school. Now it means taking courses, entire programs in a content area, and even PhD study "online" or via "distance" using the World Wide Web.

Shift from Teaching to Learning. The teacher-centered focus of education has given way to a student-centered focus upon learning (Barr & Tagg, 1995). The traditional method of content delivery, lecture, is no longer regarded as the way to impart knowledge and understanding. Rather, active learning, wherein knowledge and understanding are constructed by the learner based upon previous learning and experience, and which, concomitantly, transforms the learner in some meaningful way, is the current focus of educational innovation and is the new standard for education (Cranton, 1994). Excellence in education is now defined as assisting the student to learn knowledge, skills, or attitudes that allow them to accomplish some outcome objective. This is in marked contrast to past models of excellence wherein knowledge was presented to the student in dense and relentless ways (e.g., recall how you probably were taught neuroanatomy or physiology, or drop in on a traditional medical school lecture).

Recognition of the Need for Interdisciplinary Collaboration. The 20th century's focus upon specialization as initiated by the industrial revolution has rendered great knowledge gains, but also condemned us to insularity, segmentation, and related individualism. Given the explosion of knowledge in single fields, it is rare to find individuals who cross disciplines, fields, or areas of study. Thus, wheels are reinvented, research is unwittingly replicated, and resources are not allotted to best serve society.

These three factors will be specifically related to occupational therapy.

RELATIONSHIP TO OCCUPATIONAL THERAPY EDUCATION

Instructional Technology. Steven Gilbert (Gilbert, 2001) is a nationally recognized expert in technology as well as teaching and learning. I recently had the opportunity to hear him speak, and a key concept he imparted was about hybrids. That is, he believes that hybrid courses of study, or those that combine some aspect of live, classroom interaction coupled with some aspect of distance learning using the World Wide Web, are going to become the standard for education, just as lecture has been the standard of education for past centuries. This suggests that for occupational therapy education, hybrid forms of learning incorporating face-to-face interactions with instructors and students will be linked with or merged with other forms of educational instruction available through the World Wide Web or related technologies such as CD-ROM, streaming videos, or teleconferencing classrooms.

Shift from Teaching to Learning. Many of you may recall the movement of occupational therapy away from the term "patient" to "client" or "family centered care." Similarly, occupational therapy education is now challenged to move from a teacher-centered focus to a learner-centered focus. In fact, it has been my experience that occupational therapy is way ahead of the curve on this one, since active learning has always been a tenet of occupational therapy and easily generalizes to occupational therapy education.

Recognition of the Need for Interdisciplinary Collaboration. There is considerable literature in our field about the recognized need to collaborate across disciplines in order to provide better and more effective care to clients and their families (Conner-Kerr, Wittman, & Muzzarelli, 1998; MacKinnon & MacRae, 1996; Touchard & Berthelot, 1999; Tryssenaar, Perkins, & Brett, 1996). Yet, most occupational therapy educational programs, just like every other professional course of study, have the majority of classes in isolation from other disciplines or professions. Education as it currently operates is reinforcing individuality when teamwork and interdisciplinary education and practice are what society really needs. The need for interdisciplinary collaboration speaks to the need to evaluate and revise how we implement fieldwork education.

Considering these reflections about education and learning in occupational therapy, priorities emerge which need our attention, deliberation and action for occupational therapy education in the 21st century. They are summarized as follows:

CONSEQUENT PRIORITIES NEEDING TO BE ADDRESSED IN OCCUPATIONAL THERAPY EDUCATION FOR THE 21st CENTURY

1. *Technology in teaching and learning.* Consideration of how best to incorporate instructional technology in occupational therapy education is

critically needed. Guidelines for a variety of ways to accomplish effective use of technology in education, as well as ways to assist educators in adopting technology in education, are warranted.

2. *Assume leadership role in the demonstration of active learning.* It is my experience that the majority of occupational therapy educators use active learning in an effective manner without necessarily knowing that they are doing so. Increasing the level of understanding of educational therapy and practice, as well as understanding how occupational therapy education often epitomizes this, is appropriate.

3. *Fieldwork education: Delineation and measurement.* Fieldwork has always been an educational experience directly focusing upon student learning. Clearer articulation of how student learning in the form of fieldwork can and should occur in occupational therapy outside of medical model practice is needed. And, valid and reliable ways to measure student learning in fieldwork education are *urgently needed.* Ask any fieldwork educator.

4. *Interdisciplinary learning.* Interdisciplinary learning does not mean yet another course in the curriculum which is already overburdened. But, it does mean providing meaningful experiences for students to interact together. Given the nature and intent of the profession, a natural form for this would be service learning. Thus, guidelines for implementation of interdisciplinary service learning including occupational therapy are needed.

5. *The dignity of teaching.* Lee Shulman suggests that teaching should be a scholarly responsibility of the disciplinary community (Shulman, 1993). Thus the "Dignity of Teaching" (American Association for Higher Education, 2000) (a term used in *Campus Program Update, 2000*) may be best expressed and revered through the ways of a scholar as applied to teaching. Again, guidelines for occupational therapy education related to this are needed.

These priorities are set forth as a starting point for a concerted effort under the general rubric of the scholarship of teaching. This volume is a great example of how to increase the focus of occupational therapy education towards the scholarship of teaching. The co-editors are to be commended for this effort!

REFERENCES

American Association for Higher Education. (November, 2000). The dignity of teaching. *Campus Program Update, II,* 1.

Baldwin, R. G. (1998). Technology's impact on faculty life and work. *New Directions for Teaching and Learning, 76,* 7-21.

Barr, R. B., & Tagg, J. (1995). From teaching to learning–a new paradigm for undergraduate education. *Change, 27*(6), 12-25.

Conner-Kerr, T. A., Wittman, P., & Muzzarelli, R. (1998). Analysis of practice-role perceptions of physical therapy, occupational therapy, and speech-language therapy students. *J Allied Health, 27*(3), 128-131.

Cranton, P. (1994). *Understanding and promoting transformative learning.* San Francisco, CA: Jossey-Bass.

Gilbert, S. (2001). *Making on-line education work for students and faculty.* Paper presented at the Creighton University, School of Pharmacy and Allied Health Professions Faculty Development Workshop, Omaha, NE.

Grant, H. K. (1991). Education then and now: 1949 and 1989. *American Journal of Occupational Therapy, 45*(4), 295-299.

MacKinnon, J. L., & MacRae, N. (1996). Fostering geriatric interdisciplinary collaboration through academic education. *Phys Occup Ther Geriatr, 14*(3), 41-49.

Shulman, L. S. (1993). Teaching as a community property: Putting an end to pedagogical solitude. *Change, 25*(6), 6-7.

Touchard, B. M., & Berthelot, K. (1999). Collaborative home practice: Nursing and occupational therapy ensure appropriate medication administration. *Home Health Nurse, 17*(1), 45-51.

Tryssenaar, J., Perkins, J., & Brett, L. (1996). Undergraduate interdisciplinary education: Are we educating for future practice? *Can J Occup Ther, 63*(4), 245-251.

A Review of AOTF Programs Directed Toward Education: 1965-2000

Nedra Gillette, MEd, OTR, FAOTA

In a sense, AOTF has always been about education. Its first program was to administer and award scholarships to OT students, in both professional and technical level programs. Many of these scholarships were the result of monies bequeathed to the Foundation; some came about through early fund-raising activities.

In its next effort to serve the occupational therapy community, AOTF initiated its research programs. This was a joint effort, co-funded by AOTA. From the beginning, it was clear that research could not and did not thrive in occupational therapy because it was not incorporated as one of the core values of members of the profession. Since one's professional identity is derived through exposure to role models and by means of curriculum content and expectations, the "problem" with research (the lack thereof) lay at the feet of the profession's education system. Therefore, a large proportion of AOTF programs undertaken during the past 22 years under the auspices of "research" were directed towards faculty development.

One of the first efforts was to establish a research journal, based on the dual assumption that university faculty needed additional scholarly materials on which to base their educational strategies and that scholars in the field needed additional focused outlets for their scholarship and research. (It is interesting to note in retrospect that of the six existing formal bodies within AOTA in

Nedra Gillette is Director of Research, American Occupational Therapy Foundation.

[Haworth co-indexing entry note]: "A Review of AOTF Programs Directed Toward Education: 1965-2000." Gillette, Nedra. Co-published simultaneously in *Occupational Therapy in Health Care* (The Haworth Press, Inc.) Vol. 15, No. 1/2, 2001, pp. 215-218; and: *Education for Occupational Therapy in Health Care: Strategies for the New Millennium* (eds: Patricia Crist, and Marjorie Scaffa) The Haworth Press, Inc., 2001, pp. 215-218. Single or multiple copies of this article are available for a fee from The Haworth Document Delivery Service [1-800-HAWORTH, 9:00 a.m. - 5:00 p.m. (EST). E-mail address: getinfo@haworthpressinc.com].

215

1980 who were surveyed with regard to the need for/interest in a research journal for the field, program directors were the least enthusiastic, identifying no particular need for such a journal.) *The Occupational Therapy Journal of Research* (OTJR) was founded in 1981. Published by Slack, Inc., for the American Occupational Therapy Foundation, it has a smaller circulation than its outstanding qualities would seem to indicate. It is also more openly received and has a greater subscription list, proportionately, overseas.

The journal welcomed a new editor at the end of 2001: Dr. Carolyn Baum assumed that set of responsibilities. In preparation for her duties, she has received permission from the Foundation Board of Directors to change the name of the journal by adding a subtitle that reflects its new direction: *The Occupational Therapy Journal of Research: Occupation, Participation, and Health*. The journal will also receive an artistic face-lift in 2002 and will accept research articles that address the relationship of occupation to health, well-being, and quality of life. The journal will have three sections: developing models and theories of occupation; evidence-based practice initiatives; and the measurement of occupation and occupational performance.

Another early educational initiative is also enjoying a revision. The teaching manual, *Integrating Research into the Curriculum*, by Dr. Maralynne Mitcham, was an early and highly praised effort to provide direction to those educational programs where experienced research scholars were essentially nonexistent. This manual offered educational assignments that demonstrated the similarity between clinical judgments and those required through the research process. It provided exercises that allowed academic and clinical faculty to integrate beginning concepts of research throughout the other courses in the curriculum. In this way, students were less "shy" about research and were better able to grasp its relevance for the field as a whole.

Last summer (2001) AOTF released a newly-revised edition of this manual, designed and edited by the Foundation's Academic Development Committee. Chapters were solicited from well-known educators in the field who generously have shared their assignments, reference lists, and teaching strategies for this purpose.

The Academic Development Committee, a committee of the Research Advisory Council, has been instrumental in providing a variety of other services to the educational community in occupational therapy. Founded in 1981, the ADC has been highly responsive to identified research needs within the OT community. Research competencies originally developed in 1982 by an ad hoc AOTF committee, and done so at the request of the Representative Assembly, were revised in 1998 by the ADC. These competencies, which eventually were considered by and partially integrated into the new Standards for an Accredited Educational Program for the Occupational Therapist, can serve to guide educators in the preparation of therapists at various levels of research expertise.

Where do we go from here? AOTF is launching a new initiative, to be known as the Institute for the Study of Occupation and Health. Details are not yet worked out, but its purpose will be to support faculty development and research that help to educate the public about the impact of occupation on the health of all citizens. Higher education, scientific inquiry, and public information are the charter purposes of the American Occupational Therapy Foundation.

Our first efforts within the Institute are directed towards faculty development, in the domain of curriculum design and revision. This is a response to the needs expressed in 2000 by program directors for assistance in meeting the new Standards for an Accredited Educational Program for the Occupational Therapist, and for moving to post-baccalaureate education. Working with both AOTA and ACOTE, we have designed a series of regional workshops that respond to this need. They will be presented by a talented group of people we call "facilitators," who will work with teams of academic and clinical faculty members from a given educational program. The series is comprised of three workshops, approximately four months apart. Pre-workshop assignments will be provided online prior to each workshop. Major themes of the workshops will be: occupation as the core of practice and education; evidence-based practice as it is integrated with research courses throughout the curriculum; a set of strong links between academic and fieldwork education, and principles of curriculum design appropriate for the development of critical, independent professional judgment. Each program will develop its own unique approach to professional curriculum, as is the usual standard of ACOTE.

A second program, closely related, is being offered to five schools who competed for the opportunity to engage with a mentor in 2002 as their faculties work towards the development of a community of scholars while also attending to ACOTE requirements for the new entry-level standards. These faculties are collaborating with AOTF as we attempt to determine how and to what extent a mentoring process can effect the development of a community of scholars. This research study will use qualitative methods to document the mentoring process, the first study we know of that examines the process used by faculties in revising and upgrading professional curricula.

Other programs for the institute remain to be developed. We believe that through a focus on occupation and the utilization of the World Health Organization's new classification system, which acknowledges "activity," "participation," and "environmental context" as the basis for insuring equality for all citizens, AOTF càn promote health and well-being on a greater scale. When occupational function is at risk, or has been compromised, intervention through therapy is the logical course of action. To the extent that the public recognizes occupation as a powerful force which may be either negative or positive in its effects, the profession of occupational therapy will be recognized as the mediator of choice. Through the Institute, AOTF will continue its efforts to serve the public by developing, disseminating, and promoting knowledge about the forces of occupation and occupational therapy.

AN INVITATION

AOTF invites the educational community in occupational therapy to join us in addressing the critical issues that face us:

- the need to instill a strong positive value towards using and contributing to research in ALL entry-level students
- the need to recognize the importance of continuous testing and revision of our knowledge base and to make an effort to contribute to this process as role models for students
- the need to reflect on and critique constructively the literature of various other disciplines with regard to their theory and research as it relates to the construct of occupation, time use, participation in society, and like concepts
- the need to examine the differences between professional education and graduate education, towards the preparation of more critical thinkers
- the need to prepare graduates whose identity as therapists is more closely aligned with the "big picture," as it is represented through concepts of occupation at the societal level (such things as homelessness and unemployment; non-discriminatory policies for public transportation; aging in place; and teen-age violence, as it might be addressed through innovative models of occupational intervention)
- creative models of occupational therapy that may be applied across diverse populations of individuals, families, communities, and systems, at the prevention, intervention, and long-term rehabilitation levels.

Programs of the Institute for the Study of Occupation and Health will be directed to issues such as these. We are interested in collaborating with members of the educational community in the exploration of occupational health, and in the use of scientific inquiry to insure the significance of occupational therapy in society.

Creating Education
to Meet Health Care Predictions

Barbara Kornblau, JD, OTR/L, FAOTA

Educators cannot afford to ignore the future. Education needs a dynamic perspective that grows and adapts to meet the changing needs of society. Educators can make or break our profession's future existence. This article looks at changing trends for the future that every educator must consider, lest they be left behind in the dust.

It is certainly not news to say the population is graying. The baby boomers are transitioning from the Pepsi generation to the Geritol generation. At the same time, changes in Medicare have changed the way we provide services in almost all settings. Science and technological changes are changing the face of health care. The population has increased in diversity with the once melting-pot nation turning into a salad of multiculturalism. More children are being diagnosed with a plethora of developmental syndromes and are in need of early intervention services, which often are not covered by insurance reimbursement. More and more workers find themselves in sedentary jobs leading to repetitive trauma and other health problems.

Occupational therapy cannot claim immunity from these changes. These external changes raise many questions for the profession. What will practice look like in the future? Who will we treat? Where will we treat the older population? What will that treatment consist of? Who will pay for that treatment? How will science and technology change occupational therapy practice? What opportunities do these changes present for occupational therapy practice? How does occupational therapy assure a role in the future of treatment? How can educators facilitate occupational therapy's role in a changing future?

Barbara Kornblau is President of the American Occupational Therapy Association.

[Haworth co-indexing entry note]: "Creating Education to Meet Health Care Predictions." Kornblau, Barbara. Co-published simultaneously in *Occupational Therapy in Health Care* (The Haworth Press, Inc.) Vol. 15, No. 1/2, 2001, pp. 219-223; and: *Education for Occupational Therapy in Health Care: Strategies for the New Millennium* (eds: Patricia Crist, and Marjorie Scaffa) The Haworth Press, Inc., 2001, pp. 219-223. Single or multiple copies of this article are available for a fee from The Haworth Document Delivery Service [1-800-HAWORTH, 9:00 a.m. - 5:00 p.m. (EST). E-mail address: getinfo@haworthpressinc.com].

The occupational therapy profession must answer these questions as it plans for this future. In response to the changing external environment, occupational therapy has to proactively change to position ourselves for the future. Many of these changes are changes in how we, as a profession, view the world. Teaching these changes to position occupational therapy practitioners for future practice will fall upon the shoulders of occupational therapy educators. *Occupational therapy educators must step up to the plate to incorporate future trends into the occupational therapy curriculum and fieldwork.*

THE GRAYING POPULATION

Occupational therapy practitioners need preparation to address the needs of a growing, aging population. On the whole, baby boomers represent the most educated and most affluent group of elders this country has seen. Add to this the increased life expectancy of the baby boom generation of elders to come.

This is a generation that thrived on leisure activities. This generation went through the jogging craze, a plethora of spectator sports, and joining gyms. The baby boomers also experienced the obsession with cholesterol levels, quitting smoking, "wellness," and many other "health" fads. Baby boomers saw the forty-hour work week increase exponentially with the introduction of voice mail, cell phones, e-mail, and golf as work.

Active elders will want to remain as independent and "young" as possible for as long as possible. Their home base will lie in the community as long as possible. Occupational therapy practitioners will need to serve this population in their homes, in the community.

Occupational-based practice will play a significant role in keeping the baby boomers independent and healthy. Cone stacking will not serve this population's needs. Occupational therapy practitioners will need to assess the needs of independent retirees in their natural environments and provide intervention calculated to keep them independent and healthy. Occupational therapy practitioners need to prepare to address needs such as transition to retirement, driver training, depression, and other mental health needs, low vision, fall and injury prevention, occupational loss, occupational imbalance due to retirement, the sudden overabundance of leisure, and workplace modifications for those desiring to return to the workforce if only on a temporary basis or as volunteers.

Traditional occupational therapy courses addressing geriatrics must look to the future and prepare students to meet the needs of tomorrow's elders. Non-traditional fieldwork in community-based programs can help prepare students for the future changes to come.

CREATING INDEPENDENT, ENTREPRENEURIAL-THINKING OCCUPATIONAL THERAPISTS

Whenever I discuss the changing needs of tomorrow's elders, someone inevitably comments that Medicare doesn't cover these services. As a profession, occupational therapists need to shift their thinking from Medicare and health insurance-based reimbursement to fee-for-service-based reimbursement. To address these changing needs of seniors, and others, occupational therapy programs will need to educate and create independent, entrepreneurial-thinking occupational therapists (IETOTs).

IETOTs can go out into the community, assess needs, and develop and market occupational therapy programs to meet those needs–and they get paid for providing the services. IETOTs do not fear billing for services. IETOTs keep up on future trends and pay attention to changes in the political process that may affect their practice. IETOTs get paid for their services on a fee-for-service basis, through arrangements with corporations contracting for occupational therapy services, through grants funding, or other sources.

To create IETOTs, occupational educators must instill business values, ethics, and acumen in occupational therapy students. Students will be creating occupational therapy intervention for the future. To accomplish this, students must enter the workforce with the knowledge and skills to pursue their own dreams and visions for occupational therapy practice in all areas of occupational therapy, from womb to tomb.

SCIENCE AND TECHNOLOGICAL CHANGES

Occupational therapists need preparation to address changes in science and technology as they arise. Over the last two decades, we have witnessed technological advances improve the quantity and quality of the lives of our clients. Recent scientific and technological advances provide occupational therapy with new areas of concern. Going forward, occupational therapists will need to prepare for genetics' influences on diseases and human conditions. *To accomplish this, occupational therapy curriculum will need to address the Human Genome Project and its contribution to medical knowledge.*

The Human Genome Project identified the structure of the human genome. Researchers continue to identify more and more diseases and conditions that have a genetic basis or cause. Many occupational therapy practitioners already work with clients with conditions with genetic origins such as Alzheimer's disease, stroke, heart disease, autism, and depression. Occupational therapists will play a role in helping to identify genetic symptoms of clients' diseases or disorders and refer clients and family members for genetic testing.

The future holds what were once considered miracles. Scientists will be able to map an individual's genes and predict with near certainty the illnesses or diseases that individual will experience. However, since we know lifestyle plays a role in the emergence of many conditions of genetic origin, occupational therapy can carve out a role in lifestyle redesign to help prevent the emergence of diseases such as heart disease or other preventable or "postpone-able" diseases.

Occupational therapy educators can promote these roles by incorporating state-of-the-art scientific information into curricula and developing innovative fieldwork sites to address issues in response to the new discoveries. With this type of proactive role, educators can help assure a role for occupational therapy.

OCCUPATIONAL THERAPY AND PUBLIC HEALTH

Occupational therapists need to look at the health of populations and come to the table with the big picture of health and wellness of society in mind. Many of our themes, such as stress reduction, relaxation, falls prevention, occupation as a source of health and wellness, positive mental health, and violence prevention comport with a public health perspective. We need to develop an understanding of policy development and assert our role in public health policy formation to promote occupational therapy. *Occupational therapy educators need to incorporate public health policy information into curricula.*

As the keepers of occupation for the future, occupational therapy must promote the value of occupation as a tool for prevention and maintenance of well-being. An expanded research base, promoted by educators, can justify, for the public health community, occupation's place in injury and illness prevention, health promotion, and "wellness," giving occupational therapy a respected position in the public health community.

Many occupational therapy practitioners already function in the public health arena. The future of occupational therapy will likely move us further into the public health arena as we provide intervention to populations in total, such as groups of homeless individuals, teenagers and children at risk, and frail elders, all of whom may come from diverse populations.

CULTURAL DIVERSITY

Occupational therapy practitioners must be equipped to effectively provide treatment intervention to a wide variety of populations. Warring nations, political asylum, the global economy, and legal and illegal immigration have all changed the complexion of society. Society no longer expects individuals to assimilate into the broad American culture as it once did in past generations. Respect for one's cultural differences takes preference in contemporary society. *To meet society's need, cultural competencies must be incorporated into occupational therapy curricula at all levels so educational programs can turn out culturally competent occupational therapy practitioners.*

In order for occupational therapy practitioners to effectively provide treatment, they must become familiar with these differences. Occupational therapy practitioners or fieldwork students will likely find themselves working with clients of a culture other than their own and one with which they may lack familiarity.

Occupational therapy practitioners must also consider cultural differences in the way individuals view health, disability, and relationships with service providers. Lack of cultural competence may impede the provision of effective treatment if occupational therapy practitioners cross barriers set by cultural expectations. Further, occupational therapy practitioners must consider these cultural differences in all contexts so they may successfully market occupational therapy services and maintain co-worker harmony.

CONCLUSION

Occupational therapy practitioners need to prepare for the changing healthcare market and the changing occupational therapy market. Change happens. Occupational therapy practitioners need to adapt willingly to the change. Hospitals, nursing homes, and other medical model settings will give way to a future of non-medical model, community-based or community-built, prevention and wellness-oriented settings.

These changes bring a wealth of opportunity for occupational therapists to further practice in the community. Numerous opportunities lie in the community for geriatric programs, pediatric programs, mental health programs, and others. Practice in the community is limited only by the boundaries of one's creativity. Occupational therapy educators can play a key role in furthering this move as part of the education process and assure students will enter the marketplace with the knowledge and skills to meet the challenges that lie ahead.

Occupational Therapy Education:
At the Heart of the Profession's Future

Joseph C. Isaacs, CAE
Doris Gordon, FAOTA

The advancement of occupational therapy (OT) as a respected discipline, valued service, and desirable career choice is inextricably linked to the future of occupational therapy education. Educational programs throughout the country can feel very proud of their achievements to date. Their didactic and practice-based curricula have provided occupational therapy students with a solid grounding in the behavioral and biological sciences and occupation-based theory and research, as well as in evaluative, treatment, and implementation techniques.

These programs grew and responded well in the past to the call for greater numbers of qualified OT practitioners nationwide. Now, amid consolidation of programs, they must respond as effectively in preparing the next generation of practitioners to take advantage of evolving opportunities both within and beyond traditional practice settings and to successfully overcome obstacles in the marketplace.

The field has already begun to respond with the move to post-baccalaureate entry level to the profession. There are new ACOTE accreditation standards that reinforce the essential elements of this graduate-level education. And, ACOTE, AOTA, and AOTF have joined forces to create workshops to assist programs to make this important transition.

Joseph C. Isaacs is Executive Director of The American Occupational Therapy Association, and Doris Gordon is Director of Academic Affairs.

[Haworth co-indexing entry note]: "Occupational Therapy Education: At the Heart of the Profession's Future." Isaacs, Joseph C., and Doris Gordon. Co-published simultaneously in *Occupational Therapy in Health Care* (The Haworth Press, Inc.) Vol. 15, No. 1/2, 2001, pp. 225-229; and: *Education for Occupational Therapy in Health Care: Strategies for the New Millennium* (eds: Patricia Crist, and Marjorie Scaffa) The Haworth Press, Inc., 2001, pp. 225-229. Single or multiple copies of this article are available for a fee from The Haworth Document Delivery Service [1-800-HAWORTH, 9:00 a.m. - 5:00 p.m. (EST). E-mail address: getinfo@haworthpressinc.com].

225

FACING A LEADERSHIP CHALLENGE

Unlike the efforts to respond to the boom in demand for occupational therapists in the health and rehabilitation arenas during the 1980s and 1990s, the challenge in the new millennium is about actively promoting the contributions the profession can make to improve our rapidly changing world. Today, it is a challenge about exerting leadership, acquiring new skills and competencies, reclaiming roles, and broadening our opportunities. Though the demographic trends suggest that the demand for occupational therapy services will continue to grow, we have also learned that practitioners cannot depend on contract or employee relationships to ensure their livelihood even when need is apparent.

Managed care and government cutbacks continue to promote uncertainty in the field, motivating providers to exert greater control over referrals to occupational therapy and other professionals. Moreover, reimbursement and efficiency requirements have forced practitioners to define themselves by techniques and payment codes rather than the application of their broader problem solving skills.

As more and more occupational therapy practitioners find themselves employed within educational settings, many express similar frustrations about their scope of practice. They seldom are given the freedom to provide the wide array of services they are well capable of and, like their counterparts in more traditional physical medicine settings, feel their creativity is being stifled. How can this not be demoralizing and breed dissatisfaction? Is it any wonder, then, that fieldwork supervisors have been known to be cynical about the profession with their interns? We must restore our faith in our professional abilities, reaffirm our roots in multiple functional areas, and view those we serve more holistically.

In the mental health arena, where new resources have been devoted, can occupational therapy practitioners assert themselves in ways that reflect the profession's historical roots in psychosocial function? To effectively accomplish this, practitioners must be better prepared to assume responsibility for independent practice, serve as effective advocates for a broadened scope of practice, and apply their clinical problem solving skills and knowledge in "nontraditional" practice settings on a fee-for-service basis.

BUILDING CONFIDENCE AND PROFESSIONAL PRIDE

If one accepts the above premise, then the future avenues for applying occupational therapy seem boundless, limited only by the extent to which occupational therapy professionals are unable to make the case for their value to other stakeholders—such as consumers, payers, other providers, and policymakers. Building that capacity, as well as the confidence and professional pride needed, must begin at our educational programs. And, we at AOTA must be prepared to supplement this self-development throughout our members' careers. With the strength of these skills and competencies and a strong educational program/professional association support system behind them, occupational therapy practitioners will survive and flourish in the dynamic world they face. To enable this, the AOTA realizes that its collaboration with educational programs must be strengthened, and it is intent on doing so.

All this may sound lofty in the face of reduced educational program enrollments, tightened employment opportunities, and reimbursement and salary battles we continue to experience of late. If we are to reverse these trends and reduce our reliance on the whims of the marketplace, however, occupational therapy will have to experience a cultural change. This change is one from a profession of dependency to one of greater self-sufficiency, creativity, leadership, and more proactive personal advocacy.

Educators and practitioners are rallying in state and local communities to demonstrate that occupational therapy can be just as effective in community and public health environs, the workplace and the home as it has been in more traditional health care settings. Since "necessity is the mother of invention," there will, no doubt, be imaginative employment options created in the field if occupational therapy professionals have the tools to promote and take advantage of them.

Given this scenario, we're still faced with the dilemma of not being very well understood among consumers, insurers, certain providers, payers, policymakers, and leaders of industry. Somehow, the profession must build a better "mouse-trap," one that offers each of these publics a definition of occupational therapy that will resonate with them. This definition must be uncomplicated and convey the profession's underpinnings in high-quality education and more than 80 years of experience in helping individuals lead more productive, active lives in the face of disabling illness or injury or promoting wellness through desired lifestyle change. Occupational therapy's uniqueness lies in its capacity to create practical solutions to the challenges of living by addressing the whole person. We must reassert this boldly and proudly and advocate within the profession to once again invoke this principle in all occupational therapy practice.

ACADEMIC CROSS-FERTILIZATION WITH OTHER DISCIPLINES

Education programs are central to this strategy. We must not only produce master clinicians, but also foster creative, future-oriented independent thinkers who can contribute to advancing the profession and feel comfortable in collaborating across disciplines to do so. To instill such confidence, we must begin to partner with other disciplines at colleges and universities, when the equality of being students can foster greater acceptance of the merits of interdisciplinary team approaches involving occupational therapy.

For example, coursework and projects with students of architecture would foster their appreciation of occupational therapy in facility design, particularly in areas of disability accommodation and ergonomics. Interaction with engineering students can demonstrate to them the role of occupational therapy in ensuring optimal functionality in product research and development (e.g., assistive technologies or appliances for activities of daily living) and helping to devise well-conceived design plans.

Opportunities for direct activities with medical students will help to reinforce the appropriateness of referrals to occupational therapy practitioners and their contribution to efficacious, effective, and cost-efficient multidisciplinary approaches to patient care. Research on geographic practice variations has demonstrated that a physician's practice habits are most directly related to those developed during his or her training. Thus, one's best shot at influencing this behavior is when they are still students, interns, and residents.

Educational programs should be encouraged to build linkages to other influential professionals and disciplines and expose them to the merits of occupational therapy in what they do. These areas include, but are certainly not limited to, anthropology, business, international relations, physics, psychology and sociology, and social work. Earning the recognition from students and faculty in these other fields will help produce long-term allies and partners. It will help future occupational therapy practitioners gain the confidence to open doors in their own career advancement and lay the groundwork for future interdisciplinary opportunities.

FOSTERING BUSINESS ACUMEN, ENTREPRENEURSHIP, AND CREATIVITY

Of all the related disciplines cited above, one that educational programs must urgently infuse in their curricula is business. If occupational therapy practitioners are to have more of a say in their own destiny, then they must gain the business acumen to engage and succeed in entrepreneurial pursuits (e.g., independent practice) and help gain added economic and political clout to influence public policy and broaden their opportunities. In a recent web-based survey conducted by AOTA, in fact, more than 80 percent of the responding members called for the addition of business courses to the core occupational therapy curricula.

The typical occupational therapy student is bright, enthusiastic, and ready to conquer the world. Educational programs must provide them with a well-rounded educational experience and wide range of tools for success. We have described many in this article and encourage a milieu where students are given countless opportunities to debate and defend their views, and to demonstrate their ability to think clearly and positively on their feet. The abilities to influence others, respond to future trends, respond to objection, and convey firmly a belief in what we do are critical keys to professional success.

This is a major area where many competent students are deficient. Coming out of the classroom, they meet fierce competition, resistance to ideas, and regulations that lead them to stray from their original raison d'être. If students can assert themselves with verve, backed by the latest knowledge, oriented towards future trends and the ability to think spontaneously, they will be more apt to succeed. If they build confidence in pursuing business and interdisciplinary opportunities, they will be more apt to succeed. If they build professional pride and participate in their professional association and its efforts to define occupational therapy meaningfully to its important publics and transfer knowledge within the field, they will be more apt to succeed. And with that success, the long-held tenets of occupational therapy will be preserved and the profession's great promise will reach new heights in the years to come.

Entry Level Certification
and the Educational Community

L. Randy Strickland, EdD, OTR/L, FAOTA

The public's valuing of the importance and integrity of occupational therapy certification is an essential recognition for being a profession. Originating under the leadership of the American Occupational Therapy Association (AOTA) over seventy years ago, the occupational therapy profession has supported the use of a certification program for its practitioners in the United States. In 1987 the AOTA moved all existing certification programs for occupational therapists and occupational therapy assistants to the newly created American Occupational Therapy Certification Board (AOTCB) (Baum & Gray, 1988; AOTA, 1988; AOTA, 1989a; AOTA, 1989b). This decision has promoted the independence of the certification processes, and in 1996 AOTCB changed its name to the National Board for Certification in Occupational Therapy (NBCOT) as a reflection of its mission to evaluate the competency of occupational therapy practitioners throughout their professional careers.

The NBCOT is the independent national credentialing agency that certifies eligible persons as OCCUPATIONAL THERAPIST REGISTERED OTR® and CERTIFIED OCCUPATIONAL THERAPY ASSISTANT COTA®, hereafter referred to as OTR or COTA. Our mission of serving the public interest includes providing high standards for the certification of occupational therapy practitioners. Certification by NBCOT is a symbol of quality–to the practitioner, the employer, and the client. In today's continually changing

L. Randy Strickland is President, National Board for Certification in Occupational Therapy, and Professor and Chair, Auerbach School of Occupational Therapy, Spalding University, Louisville, KY.

[Haworth co-indexing entry note]: "Entry Level Certification and the Educational Community." Strickland, L. Randy. Co-published simultaneously in *Occupational Therapy in Health Care* (The Haworth Press, Inc.) Vol. 15, No. 1/2, 2001, pp. 231-235; and: *Education for Occupational Therapy in Health Care: Strategies for the New Millennium* (eds: Patricia Crist, and Marjorie Scaffa) The Haworth Press, Inc., 2001, pp. 231-235. Single or multiple copies of this article are available for a fee from The Haworth Document Delivery Service [1-800-HAWORTH, 9:00 a.m. - 5:00 p.m. (EST). E-mail address: getinfo@haworthpressinc.com].

health and human services environments our certification programs serve as a constant and consistent benchmark for the public and profession. Certification represents the adherence to high principles, which help to ensure the provision of quality services and protect the integrity and value of occupational therapy programming and the profession. To effectively anticipate and plan for changes in the practice environment, NBCOT continually engages in a myriad of collaborative activities with the practice, regulatory, educational, and professional association communities.

Since the inception of certification within the profession, educators have been keenly interested in these processes. Our profession has been efficient and proactive in the identification of the requirements for initial certification as an occupational therapy practitioner. To be eligible to sit for the certification examination, a candidate must have successfully completed an educational program that is accredited by the Accreditation Council for Occupational Therapy Education and must not have a criminal background that would prevent them from being certified as a safe, competent practitioner. Understanding the role of NBCOT is important since this organization's mission is to serve the public interest. This role includes the development and implementation of certification programs which assure that qualified and appropriately credentialed practitioners deliver occupational therapy services. Occupational therapy state regulatory boards use the NBCOT certification examination as a major criteria for credentialing practitioners.

CERTIFICATION EXAMINATION

The creation of certification examinations for both the OTR and COTA levels is a multifaceted process involving educators and practitioners. Each examination must be reflective of the validated expectations of entry-level OTRs and COTAs in practice settings. The purpose of our most recent practice analysis in 1997–the *National Study of Occupational Therapy Practice* (NBCOT, 1997)–was to identify the tasks associated with current occupational therapy practice and to delineate the knowledge and skills necessary to perform those tasks. The practice analysis is the foundation upon which NBCOT establishes the content validity and test specifications or content outlines for the OTR and COTA examinations.

The passing score established for each of the OTR and COTA examinations has been set so that candidates who demonstrate "just enough knowledge and skills to merit certification" pass. All NBCOT certification examinations are criterion-referenced, which means that the passing score is based on an *absolute* level of mastery required to pass the examination. The percentage of candidates passing the examination is *not* determined prior to the test administration. Our procedure follows recommended testing procedures of the American Educational Research Association, American Psychological Association and the National Council on Measurement in Education (1999), and sets a passing score based on content specialists' judgments of the expected test performance of candidates who are minimally competent to practice at entry-level. The use of a criterion-referenced standard ensures that the level of knowledge and skill required to pass the examination is constant across test administrations. Successful completion of the NBCOT certification examination is the means of assuring the public, and, ultimately, consumers of occupational therapy services, that the OTR or COTA has met an established measure of initial practice competence.

The development of the 1997 practice analysis is a direct result of the active participation of over 3,700 practitioners and educators throughout the nation. Every effort was made to promote the inclusion of diverse practice settings and practitioners. The survey data provided critical information for academic and fieldwork educators relative to current practice and the focus of future certification examinations commencing in 2000. For example, the study found that therapists are more involved in supervision and the evaluation/program planning process, and assistants are devoting a larger amount of time in providing direct interventions. Additionally, the data revealed that two newly defined areas including the provision of population-based services and the use of occupation as an essential foundation of practice were emerging (Dunn & Cada, 1998). These findings and others directly impacted the actual examination outline, its weightings on the different content areas, and the development of specific test items requiring knowledge of daily practice requirements. The NBCOT certification examinations must be based upon current practice.

The actual test items on each examination are compiled by the NBCOT Certification Examination Development Committee (CEDC) and include practice-based questions prepared from item writers nationwide. CEDC membership includes both OTRs and COTAs who work on separate subcommittees for each respective examination level. All individuals involved in the development of the examination recognize the high stakes of the examination outcome for each potential candidate; they are equally cognizant of their tremendous responsibility in preparing a fair examination that serves the public interest and ensures that minimally competent occupational therapy practitioners are credentialed by NBCOT.

Academic Curriculum and NBCOT Interaction

Educational program faculty and fieldwork educators are keenly interested in the certification exam development and program graduate outcomes. This practice-based examination provides educators with a "window" to study their curricula and consider developments in practice. Also, academic programs may be held accountable for certification exam outcomes by the administration in their university or college. While a program may be accredited, having difficulty with a pattern of recurring numbers of graduates who do not successfully pass the certification exam may be viewed as problematic and an indicator of educational program quality by external stakeholders.

Educators and candidates may query as to why the certification examination standards and the academic program accreditation standards are not the same. In reality, this difference and separation is beneficial to the consumer, the educational program, student, and the profession. The academic accreditation of an occupational therapy program certainly may consider candidate performance on the certification examination as one outcome indicator; however, the rigor of an academic program generally reaches beyond a basic premise of the certification exam which establishes minimal competence for practice. An inspection of the NBCOT examination outlines for the OTR and COTA reveals each area is also considered in ACOTE standards. This dynamic balancing between education and certification standards promotes the broad preparation of candidates who can meet the varied needs of clients in current and future practice environments. Successfully passing the certification examination demonstrates that the candidate has demonstrated a minimum level of knowledge on a practice-based examination to safely deliver occupational therapy services; the candidate's academic preparation provides a broad foundation for practice challenges and the further enhancement and development of the profession.

NBCOT recognizes that there will always be challenges in the design and implementation of a comprehensive certification program for occupational therapy practitioners. The Board has posed thought-provoking questions regarding certification and continues to seek the input of the public, practitioners, educators, regulators, and professional associations in the ongoing design of our certification programs. Our Board affirms its mission and continued commitment to serve the public interest, which ultimately supports the integrity, value, and stability of the occupational therapy profession.

REFERENCES

American Educational Research Association, American Psychological Association, National Council on Measurement in Education. (1999). *Standards for Educational and Psychological Testing*. Washington DC: American Educational Research Association.

American Occupational Therapy Association. (1988, April). *Agreement for AOTCB Incorporation*. Rockville, MD: Author.

American Occupational Therapy Association. (1989a, June). *AOTA/AOTCB Transfer Agreement*. Rockville, MD: Author.

American Occupational Therapy Association. (1989b, June). *AOTA/AOTCB Transfer & Service Agreement Amendment*. Rockville, MD: Author.

Baum, C. M., & Gray, M. S. (1988). Certification: Serving the public interest. *American Journal of Occupational Therapy, 42* (2), 77-79.

Dunn, W., & Cada, E. (1998). The national occupational therapy practice analysis: Finding and implications for competence. *American Journal of Occupational Therapy, 52* (9), 721-728.

National Board for Certification in Occupational Therapy, Inc. (1997). *National Study of Occupational Therapy Practice*. Gaithersburg MD: NBCOT.

Index

T - #0512 - 101024 - C0 - 212/152/14 - PB - 9780789016874 - Gloss Lamination